T0263115

Necrotizing Enterocolitis

Editor

MICHAEL S. CAPLAN

CLINICS IN PERINATOLOGY

www.perinatology.theclinics.com

Consulting Editor
LUCKY JAIN

March 2019 • Volume 46 • Number 1

ELSEVIER

1600 John F. Kennedy Boulevard • Suite 1800 • Philadelphia, Pennsylvania, 19103-2899

http://www.theclinics.com

CLINICS IN PERINATOLOGY Volume 46, Number 1
March 2019 ISSN 0095-5108, ISBN-13: 978-0-323-65534-7

Editor: Kerry Holland
Developmental Editor: Casey Potter

Clinics in Perinatology (ISSN 0095-5108) is published quarterly by Elsevier Inc., 360 Park Avenue South, New York, NY 10010-1710. Months of issue are March, June, September, and December. Business and Editorial Offices: 1600 John F. Kennedy Blvd., Ste. 1800, Philadelphia, PA 19103-2899. Customer Service Office: 3251 Riverport Lane, Maryland Heights, MO 63043. Periodicals postage paid at New York, NY and additional mailing offices. Subscription prices are $309.00 per year (US individuals), $578.00 per year (US institutions), $365.00 per year (Canadian individuals), $708.00 per year (Canadian institutions), $435.00 per year (international individuals), $708.00 per year (international institutions), $100.00 per year (US students), and $195.00 per year (Canadian and international students). International air speed delivery is included in all Clinics subscription prices. All prices are subject to change without notice. **POSTMASTER:** Send address changes to *Clinics in Perinatology*, Elsevier Health Sciences Division, Subscription Customer Service, 3251 Riverport Lane, Maryland Heights, MO 63043. **Customer Service: Telephone: 1-800-654-2452** (U.S. and Canada); **1-314-447-8871** (outside U.S. and Canada); **Fax: 1-314-447-8029. E-mail: journalscustomerservice-usa@elsevier.com** (for print support); **journalsonlinesupport-usa@elsevier.com** (for online support).

Reprints. For copies of 100 or more, of articles in this publication, please contact the Commercial Reprints Department, Elsevier Inc., 360 Park Avenue South, New York, NY 10010-1710. Tel. 212-633-3874; Fax: 212-633-3820; E-mail: reprints@elsevier.com.

Clinics in Perinatology is also pubilshed in Spanish by McGraw-Hill Interamericana Editores S.A., P.O. Box 5-237, 06500 Mexico D.F., Mexico.

Clinics in Perinatology is covered in *MEDLINE/PubMed (Index Medicus) Current Contents, Excepta Medica, BIOSIS and ISI/BIOMED.*

Contributors

CONSULTING EDITOR

LUCKY JAIN, MD, MBA
George W. Brumley Jr Professor and Chair, Emory University School of Medicine, Department of Pediatrics, Chief Academic Officer, Children's Healthcare of Atlanta, Executive Director, Emory and Children's Pediatric Institute, Atlanta, Georgia, USA

EDITOR

MICHAEL S. CAPLAN, MD
Chairman, Department of Pediatrics, Chief Scientific Officer, Research Institute, NorthShore University HealthSystem, Evanston Hospital, Evanston, Illinois, USA; Clinical Professor of Pediatrics, Pritzker School of Medicine, The University of Chicago, Chicago, Illinois, USA

AUTHORS

CHERYL BATTERSBY, MBChB, FRCPCH, PhD
Senior Lecturer in Neonatal Medicine, Section of Neonatal Medicine, Department of Medicine, Imperial College London, London, United Kingdom

GAIL E. BESNER, MD
Chief, Department of Pediatric Surgery, H. William Clatworthy, Jr., Professor of Surgery, Center for Perinatal Research, The Research Institute, Nationwide Children's Hospital, The Ohio State University College of Medicine, Columbus, Ohio, USA

MICHAEL S. CAPLAN, MD
Chairman, Department of Pediatrics, Chief Scientific Officer, Research Institute, NorthShore University HealthSystem, Evanston Hospital, Evanston, Illinois, USA; Clinical Professor of Pediatrics, Pritzker School of Medicine, The University of Chicago, Chicago, Illinois, USA

BENJAMIN D. CARR, MD
House Officer, Department of Surgery, C.S. Mott Children's Hospital, University of Michigan, Ann Arbor, Michigan, USA

ERIKA C. CLAUD, MD
Professor, Neonatology, Department of Pediatrics, The University of Chicago, Chicago, Illinois, USA

C. MICHAEL COTTEN, MD, MHS
Professor, Department of Pediatrics, Division of Neonatal-Perinatal Medicine, Duke University School of Medicine, Durham, North Carolina, USA

BARRETT CROMEENS, DO
Surgical Research Fellow, Department of Pediatric Surgery, Center for Perinatal Research, The Research Institute, Nationwide Children's Hospital, The Ohio State University College of Medicine, Columbus, Ohio, USA

BRANDY L. FROST, MD
Clinical Assistant Professor, Department of Pediatrics, NorthShore University HealthSystem, Pritzker School of Medicine, The University of Chicago, Evanston, Illinois, USA

SAMIR K. GADEPALLI, MD, MBA
Assistant Professor of Pediatric Surgery and Surgical Critical Care, Section of Pediatric Surgery, Department of Surgery, C.S. Mott Children's Hospital, University of Michigan, Ann Arbor, Michigan, USA

NANCY A. GAROFALO, PhD, APRN, NNP
Neonatal Nurse Practitioner, Department of Pediatrics, NorthShore University HealthSystem, Evanston Hospital, Evanston, Illinois, USA; Senior Clinician Researcher, Pritzker School of Medicine, The University of Chicago, Chicago, Illinois, USA

SHEILA M. GEPHART, PhD, RN
Associate Professor, Community and Health Systems Science Division, College of Nursing, The University of Arizona, Tucson, Arizona, USA

GREGORY P. GOLDSTEIN, MD
Department of Pediatrics, Stanford University School of Medicine, Palo Alto, California, USA

MISTY GOOD, MD, MS
Division of Newborn Medicine, Assistant Professor, Departments of Pediatrics, and Pathology and Immunology, Washington University School of Medicine, St. Louis Children's Hospital, St Louis, Missouri, USA

CASSANDRA D. JOSEPHSON, MD
Center for Transfusion and Cellular Therapies, Departments of Pathology and Laboratory Medicine, and Pediatrics, Emory University School of Medicine, Atlanta, Georgia, USA

CHRISTINA S. KIM, MD
Fellow, Neonatology, Department of Pediatrics, The University of Chicago, Chicago, Illinois, USA

JAE H. KIM, MD, PhD
Professor of Clinical Pediatrics, Director, SPIN Program, Scientific Director, San Diego Mothers' Milk Bank, Divisions of Neonatology and Gastroenterology, Hepatology and Nutrition, University of California, San Diego, Rady Children's Hospital of San Diego, La Jolla, California, USA

BELGACEM MIHI, DVM, PhD
Division of Newborn Medicine, Departments of Pediatrics, and Pathology and Immunology, Washington University School of Medicine, St Louis, Missouri, USA

NEENA MODI, MBChB, FRCP, FRCPCH, MD
Professor of Neonatal Medicine, Section of Neonatal Medicine, Department of Medicine, Imperial College London, London, United Kingdom

KATHERINE M. NEWNAM, PhD, RN, CPNP, NNP-BC, IBCLE
Assistant Professor, School of Nursing, The University of Tennessee, Knoxville, Knoxville, Tennessee, USA

RAVI MANGAL PATEL, MD, MSc
Division of Neonatal-Perinatal Medicine, Department of Pediatrics, Emory University School of Medicine, Children's Healthcare of Atlanta, Atlanta, Georgia, USA

TERRANCE M. RAGER, MD
Surgical Research Fellow, Department of Pediatric Surgery, Center for Perinatal Research, The Research Institute, Nationwide Children's Hospital, The Ohio State University College of Medicine, Columbus, Ohio, USA

VIVEK SAROHA, MD, PhD
Division of Neonatal-Perinatal Medicine, Department of Pediatrics, Emory University School of Medicine, Children's Healthcare of Atlanta, Atlanta, Georgia, USA

RITA D. SHELBY, MD
Surgical Research Fellow, Department of Pediatric Surgery, Center for Perinatal Research, The Research Institute, Nationwide Children's Hospital, The Ohio State University College of Medicine, Columbus, Ohio, USA

KARL G. SYLVESTER, MD
Professor of Surgery and Pediatrics, Department of Surgery, Stanford University School of Medicine, Palo Alto, California, USA

Contents

Foreword: We Need to Stamp Out Necrotizing Enterocolitis   xv

Lucky Jain

Preface: Improving Outcomes Due to Neonatal Necrotizing Enterocolitis   xvii

Michael S. Caplan

Biomarker Discovery and Utility in Necrotizing Enterocolitis   1

Gregory P. Goldstein and Karl G. Sylvester

Necrotizing enterocolitis (NEC) is a devastating disease of prematurity, with no current method for early diagnosis. Diagnosis is particularly challenging, frequently occurring after the disease has progressed to the point of significant and often irreversible intestinal damage. Biomarker research has tremendous potential to advance clinical management of NEC and our understanding of its pathogenesis. This review discusses the need for novel biomarkers in NEC management, evaluates studies investigating such biomarkers, and explains the difficulties associated with translating biomarker discovery into clinical use.

Challenges in Advancing Necrotizing Enterocolitis Research   19

Cheryl Battersby and Neena Modi

Progressing necrotizing enterocolitis research is difficult because the disease is variable in presentation, there are difficulties in making a precise diagnosis, a reliable agreed case-definition is currently lacking, and there is a paucity of preclinical research to identify etiologic targets. The major challenges of the cost of clinical trials and need for long-term outcome ascertainment could be eased through incorporation of novel randomization approaches and data collection into routine care, and collaboration between public-sector and industry funders.

Necrotizing Enterocolitis Pathophysiology: How Microbiome Data Alter Our
Understanding   29

Christina S. Kim and Erika C. Claud

Necrotizing enterocolitis is a major cause of mortality and morbidity in the preterm infant population. The gut microbiome is of particular interest in research surrounding necrotizing enterocolitis, because variations in the intestinal microbiota seem to correlate with the risk of inflammation and disease. Recent advances in non–culture-based genomic sequencing have also allowed for more intricate analyses of the intestinal microbiome. Its evolution seems to be influenced by intrauterine and extra-uterine factors, ranging from antenatal antibiotic exposure to type of enteral feeds. Ultimately, these alterations in the gut microbiome have the potential to result in devastating diseases like necrotizing enterocolitis.

Closing the Gap Between Recommended and Actual Human Milk Use for Fragile Infants: What Will It Take to Overcome Disparities?   39

Sheila M. Gephart and Katherine M. Newnam

This article describes the components of human milk and their value to reduce risk for necrotizing enterocolitis, disparities in access to human milk, potential relationships to care practices within the neonatal intensive care unit, and ways to overcome the disparity.

Influence of Growth Factors on the Development of Necrotizing Enterocolitis   51

Rita D. Shelby, Barrett Cromeens, Terrance M. Rager, and Gail E. Besner

Growth factors have important roles in gastrointestinal tract development, maintenance, and response to injury. Various experiments have been used to demonstrate growth factor influence in multiple disease processes. These studies demonstrated enhancement of mucosal proliferation, intestinal motility, immune modulation, and many other beneficial effects. Select growth factors, including epidermal growth factor and heparin-binding epidermal growth factor like growth factor, demonstrate some beneficial effects in experimental and clinical intestinal injury demonstrated in necrotizing enterocolitis. The roles of glucagon-like peptide 2, insulin-like growth factor 1, erythropoietin, growth hormone, and hepatocyte growth factor in necrotizing enterocolitis are summarized in this article.

Can Fish Oil Reduce the Incidence of Necrotizing Enterocolitis by Altering the Inflammatory Response?   65

Brandy L. Frost and Michael S. Caplan

Necrotizing enterocolitis (NEC) is a devastating bowel necrosis that predominantly affects preterm infants and is characterized by an imbalance toward a proinflammatory state. Fish oil or omega-3 long-chain polyunsaturated fatty acids have the potential to modulate inflammation. In this article, the authors examine the evidence in support of fish oil supplementation to alter the inflammatory response and potentially reduce the risk of NEC.

Oropharyngeal Mother's Milk: State of the Science and Influence on Necrotizing Enterocolitis   77

Nancy A. Garofalo and Michael S. Caplan

Oropharyngeal administration of mother's own milk—placing drops of milk directly onto the neonate's oral mucosa—may serve to (ex utero) mimic the protective effects of amniotic fluid for the extremely low birth weight infant; providing protection against necrotizing enterocolitis. This article presents current evidence to support biological plausibility for the use of OroPharyngeal Therapy with Mother's Own Milk (OPT-MOM) as an immunomodulatory therapy; an adjunct to enteral feeds of mother's milk administered via a nasogastric or orogastric tube. Current methods and techniques are reviewed, published evidence to guide clinical practice will be presented, and controversies in practice will be addressed.

Does Surgical Management Alter Outcome in Necrotizing Enterocolitis? 89

Benjamin D. Carr and Samir K. Gadepalli

Necrotizing enterocolitis occurs in 14% of infants less than 1000 g. Preoperative management varies widely, and the only absolute indication for surgery is pneumoperitoneum. Multiple biomarkers and scoring systems are under investigation, but clinical practice is still largely driven by surgeon judgment. Outcomes in panintestinal disease are poor, and multiple creative approaches are used to preserve bowel length. Overall, recovery is complicated in the short and long term. Major sequelae are stricture, short gut syndrome, and neurodevelopmental impairment. Resolving controversies in surgical necrotizing enterocolitis care requires multicenter collaboration for centralized data and tissue repositories, benchmarking, and carrying out prospective randomized controlled trials.

Epidemiology of Necrotizing Enterocolitis: New Considerations Regarding the Influence of Red Blood Cell Transfusions and Anemia 101

Vivek Saroha, Cassandra D. Josephson, and Ravi Mangal Patel

This article summarizes available evidence on the relationship between red blood cell transfusion and anemia, and necrotizing enterocolitis (NEC). We review recent studies that highlight the uncertainty of the effect of red blood cell transfusion on NEC and the potential role of anemia. We also discuss potential pathophysiologic effects of both red blood cell transfusion and anemia and highlight strategies to prevent anemia and red blood cell transfusion. We also discuss ongoing randomized trials that are likely to provide important new evidence to guide red blood cell transfusion practices.

Role of Abdominal US in Diagnosis of NEC 119

Jae H. Kim

Current assessment for and diagnosis of necrotizing enterocolitis (NEC) remain inadequate. The introduction of interrogating bowel with ultrasound when NEC is suspected or when NEC has occurred presents greater opportunity to characterize the physical changes that have occurred in the bowel wall structures. The evaluation of bowel by ultrasound has been shown to have high specificity for bowel necrosis. There are current barriers in adoption of these techniques because they have not been integrated into routine diagnostic imaging and are not well incorporated in neonatal medicine.

Modifiable Risk Factors in Necrotizing Enterocolitis 129

C. Michael Cotten

Multicenter groups have reported reductions in the incidence of necrotizing enterocolitis (NEC) among preterm infants over the past 2 decades. These large-scale prevalence studies have coincided with reports from multicenter consortia and single centers of modifications in practice using quality-improvement techniques aimed at either reducing NEC risk specifically or reducing risk of mortality and multiple morbidities associated with extreme prematurity. The modifications in practice have been based on mechanistic studies, epidemiologic association data, and clinical trials. Recent reports from centers modifying practice to reduce NEC are reviewed and select modified/modifiable practices discussed.

Impact of Toll-Like Receptor 4 Signaling in Necrotizing Enterocolitis: The State of the Science   **145**

Belgacem Mihi and Misty Good

Necrotizing enterocolitis (NEC) remains a leading cause of preterm infant mortality. NEC is multifactorial and believed a consequence of intestinal immaturity, microbial dysbiosis, and an exuberant inflammatory response. Over the past decade, exaggerated Toll-like receptor 4 (TLR4) activity in the immature intestine of preterm neonates emerged as an inciting event preceding NEC. Increased TLR4 signaling in epithelial cells results in the initiation of an uncontrolled immune response and destruction of the mucosal barrier. This article discusses the state of the science of the molecular mechanisms involved in TLR4-mediated inflammation during NEC and the development of new therapeutic strategies to prevent NEC.

PROGRAM OBJECTIVE
The goal of *Clinics in Perinatology* is to keep practicing perinatologists, neonatologists, obstetricians, practicing physicians and residents up to date with current clinical practice in perinatology by providing timely articles reviewing the state of the art in patient care.

TARGET AUDIENCE
Perinatologists, neonatologists, obstetricians, practicing physicians, residents and healthcare professionals who provide patient care utilizing findings from *Clinics in Perinatology*.

LEARNING OBJECTIVES
Upon completion of this activity, participants will be able to:
1. Review available evidence on the relationship between red blood cell transfusion, anemia and necrotizing enterocolitis (NEC).
2. Discuss new therapeutic strategies to prevent NEC.
3. Recognize current evidence to support biological plausibility for the use of OPT-MOM as an immunomodulatory therapy.

ACCREDITATION
The Elsevier Office of Continuing Medical Education (EOCME) is accredited by the Accreditation Council for Continuing Medical Education (ACCME) to provide continuing medical education for physicians.

The EOCME designates this enduring material for a maximum of 15 *AMA PRA Category 1 Credit*(s)™. Physicians should claim only the credit commensurate with the extent of their participation in the activity.

All other health care professionals requesting continuing education credit for this enduring material will be issued a certificate of participation.

DISCLOSURE OF CONFLICTS OF INTEREST
The EOCME assesses conflict of interest with its instructors, faculty, planners, and other individuals who are in a position to control the content of CME activities. All relevant conflicts of interest that are identified are thoroughly vetted by EOCME for fair balance, scientific objectivity, and patient care recommendations. EOCME is committed to providing its learners with CME activities that promote improvements or quality in healthcare and not a specific proprietary business or a commercial interest.

The planning committee, staff, authors and editors listed below have identified no financial relationships or relationships to products or devices they or their spouse/life partner have with commercial interest related to the content of this CME activity:
Cheryl Battersby, MBChB, MRCPCH, FRCPCH, PhD; Gail E. Besner, MD; Benjamin D. Carr, MD; Erika C. Claud, MD; C. Michael Cotten, MD, MHS; Barrett Cromeens, DO; Samir K. Gadepalli, MD, MBA; Nancy A. Garofalo, PhD, APRN, NNP; Sheila M. Gephart, PhD, RN; Gregory P. Goldstein, MD; Misty Good, MD, MS; Kerry Holland; Lucky Jain; Cassandra D. Josephson, MD; Alison Kemp; Christina S. Kim, MD; Belgacem Mihi, DVM, PhD; Neena Modi, MBChB, FRCP, FRCPCH, MD; Swaminathan Nagarajan; Katherine M. Newnam, PhD, RN, CPNP, NNP-BC, IBCLE; Ravi Mangal Patel, MD, MSc; Terrance M. Rager, MD; Vivek Saroha, MD, PhD; Rita D. Shelby, MD; Karl G. Sylvester, MD.

The planning committee, staff, authors and editors listed below have identified financial relationships or relationships to products or devices they or their spouse/life partner have with commercial interest related to the content of this CME activity:
Michael S. Caplan, MD: participates in speakers' bureau for Mead Johnson & Company, LLC and is a consultant/advisor for Leadiant Biosciences, Ltd.
Brandy L. Frost, MD: receives research support from Mead Johnson & Company, LLC and Leadiant Biosciences, Ltd.
Jae H. Kim, MD, PhD: is a consultant/advisor for Medela LLC, Ferring Pharmaceuticals, Alcresta Therapeutics, Inc. and has participated in speakers' bureau for Mead Johnson & Company, LLC and Abbott.

UNAPPROVED/OFF-LABEL USE DISCLOSURE
The EOCME requires CME faculty to disclose to the participants:
1. When products or procedures being discussed are off-label, unlabelled, experimental, and/or investigational (not US Food and Drug Administration [FDA] approved); and
2. Any limitations on the information presented, such as data that are preliminary or that represent ongoing research, interim analyses, and/or unsupported opinions. Faculty may discuss information about

pharmaceutical agents that is outside of FDA-approved labelling. This information is intended solely for CME and is not intended to promote off-label use of these medications. If you have any questions, contact the medical affairs department of the manufacturer for the most recent prescribing information.

TO ENROLL

To enroll in the *Clinics in Perinatology* Continuing Medical Education program, call customer service at 1-800-654-2452 or sign up online at http://www.theclinics.com/home/cme. The CME program is available to subscribers for an additional annual fee of 244.40 USD.

METHOD OF PARTICIPATION

In order to claim credit, participants must complete the following:

1. Complete enrolment as indicated above.
2. Read the activity.
3. Complete the CME Test and Evaluation. Participants must achieve a score of 70% on the test. All CME Tests and Evaluations must be completed online.

CME INQUIRIES/SPECIAL NEEDS

For all CME inquiries or special needs, please contact elsevierCME@elsevier.com.

CLINICS IN PERINATOLOGY

FORTHCOMING ISSUES

June 2019
Perinatal Pharmacology
Jonathan M. Davis and
Errol Norwitz, *Editors*

September 2019
Hospital Medicine and Clinical Education
Nancy Spector, *Editor*

December 2019
Anesthesia, Sedation, and Pain Control
Shannon Hamrick and Caleb H. Ing,
Editors

RECENT ISSUES

December 2018
Diagnosis and Management of Pediatric ENT Conditions
Steven L. Goudy, *Editor*

September 2018
Long-Term Neurodevelopmental Outcomes of NICU Graduates
Ira Adams Chapman and Sara B. DeMauro, *Editors*

June 2018
Perinatal Interventions to Improve Neonatal Outcomes
Ravi Mangal Patel and Tracy A. Manuck, *Editors*

SERIES OF RELATED INTEREST

Pediatric Clinics
https://www.pediatric.theclinics.com/

THE CLINICS ARE AVAILABLE ONLINE!
Access your subscription at:
www.theclinics.com

Foreword

We Need to Stamp Out Necrotizing Enterocolitis

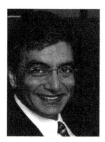

Lucky Jain, MD, MBA
Consulting Editor

Few conditions in the neonatal intensive care unit (NICU) provoke the level of fear, helplessness, and despair as does necrotizing enterocolitis (NEC). While our understanding of several aspects of the disease has improved over time, strategies for early diagnosis and treatment have remained largely elusive. A recent study[1] evaluating the incidence of NEC in high-income countries found a nearly fourfold difference (2% to 7%) in the rate of NEC among infants born less than 32 weeks' gestation and a staggering fivefold difference (5% to 22%) among those with birth weight less than 1000 grams. While some of these differences may be due to inconsistencies in definitions used, it is hard to deny that many NICUs (and nations) do far better than others in reducing the scourge of this disease. There are modifiable risk factors and differences in clinical practices such as feeding practices, use of human milk, and antibiotic stewardship, that directly impact NEC and need to be addressed.[2]

One such practice variation that cannot be ignored is in the use of human milk. Human milk feeding has been credited with the most consistent reduction in NEC in premature infants, and recent trials utilizing exclusive human milk feeds add strength to this promise. In situations where mother's own milk is not available, use of donor breast milk (compared with preterm formula) decreases the risk of NEC.[3] Yet, use of human milk in preterm infants is inconsistent and far from satisfactory. There are also wide variations among centers in feeding practices, including feeding initiation, advancement, and time to full feeds.

Deficiencies in the neonatal immune system and host defenses, particularly in the preterm infant, are well known. Human milk is naturally enriched with many agents that can modulate the neonate's immature responses to pathogens. Lactoferrin has emerged as an important component in human and bovine milk with several biologic properties that can be beneficial to the newborn (**Fig. 1**).[4] This and other promising

Clin Perinatol 46 (2019) xv–xvi
https://doi.org/10.1016/j.clp.2018.12.002
0095-5108/19/© 2018 Published by Elsevier Inc.

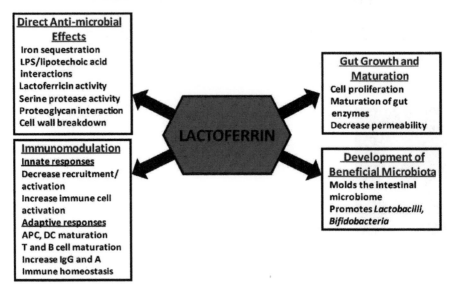

Fig. 1. Functions of lactoferrin in neonatal host defense. APC, antigen-presenting cell; IgG, immunoglobulin G; LPS, lipopolysaccharide. (*From* Telang S. Lactoferrin: a critical player in neonatal host defense. Nutrients 2018;10(9):4; with permission.)

approaches such as the use of probiotics still await more definitive data and are yet to become the standard of care.

Dr Caplan and his colleagues have done a great job in covering these and many other important topics in this issue of the *Clinics in Perinatology* . As always, I am grateful to Kerry Holland and Casey Potter at Elsevier and to you, our readers, for another great year of sharing information and advancing knowledge.

Lucky Jain, MD, MBA
Department of Pediatrics
Emory University School of Medicine
Children's Healthcare of Atlanta
1760 Haygood Drive, W409
Atlanta, GA 30322, USA

E-mail address:
ljain@emory.edu

REFERENCES

1. Battersby C, Santhalingam T, Costeloe K, et al. Incidence of neonatal nectrotising enterocolitis in high-income countries: a systematic review. Arch Dis Child Fetal Neonatal Ed 2018;103:F182–9.
2. Nino DF, Sodhi CP, Hackam DJ. Necrotizing enterocolitis: new insights into patho-genesis and mechanisms. Nat Rev Gastroenterol Hepatol 2016;13:590–600.
3. Kantorowska A, Wei JC, Cohen RS, et al. Impact of donor breast milk availability on breast milk use and necrotizing enterocolitis rates. Pediatrics 2016;137(3):e20153123.
4. Telang S. Lactoferrin: a critical player in neonatal host defense. Nutrients 2018;10(9):1228.

Preface

Improving Outcomes Due to Neonatal Necrotizing Enterocolitis

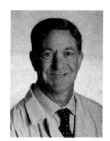

Michael S. Caplan, MD
Editor

The incidence of necrotizing enterocolitis (NEC) has only marginally improved over the last 10 years, yet many new advances have been developed that might further reduce the morbidity and mortality of this dreaded disease. In this issue of *Clinics in Perinatology*, several provocative articles are presented that address the state-of-the-art of NEC prevention, pathophysiology, and treatment, and in many instances, the authors propose novel approaches that may impact this overwhelming disease burden. For example, Dr Modi discusses the current state of NEC research and proposes approaches to reduce morbidity and mortality, while Dr Cotten describes modifiable risk factors that already may be influencing the prevalence of NEC. Additional articles focus on biomarker discovery, microbiome data, and the influence of packed red blood cell transfusions, and these all provide the context for better diagnosis and prevention of the disease. Provocative new observations suggest that fish oils, oral mother's milk supplementation, human milk, human toll-like receptor antagonists, and a variety of growth factors may be used to prevent the initiation of NEC in some patients, and these articles review the current understanding of these interesting pathways. Finally, efficient diagnosis with ultrasound techniques and subsequent surgical management for advanced NEC cases are described, and these articles frame the current clinical thinking that may currently improve outcomes. In summary, this issue provides novel

Clin Perinatol 46 (2019) xvii–xviii
https://doi.org/10.1016/j.clp.2018.12.001
0095-5108/19/© 2018 Published by Elsevier Inc.

insight into the future of NEC prevention and management and suggests provocative approaches that could move the dial dramatically in the not too distant future.

Michael S. Caplan, MD
Department of Pediatrics
North Shore University Health System
Evanston Hospital
2650 Ridge Avenue
Evanston, IL 60201, USA

E-mail address:
mcaplan@northshore.org

Biomarker Discovery and Utility in Necrotizing Enterocolitis

Gregory P. Goldstein, MD[a], Karl G. Sylvester, MD[b],*

KEYWORDS

- Necrotizing enterocolitis • Biomarker discovery • Biomarker • Diagnosis
- Pathogenesis

KEY POINTS

- Biomarker research has tremendous potential to advance clinical management of necrotizing enterocolitis (NEC) and to deepen our understanding of its pathogenesis.
- A variety of biomarkers have been shown to perform with good sensitivity or specificity for NEC diagnosis including IAIP, hydrogen excretion, VOCs, fecal microbiota analysis, and proteomic approaches, but each of these require further validity testing.
- Overall, there is a need for multicenter validation studies of already existing NEC biomarkers.

NEED FOR BIOMARKER DISCOVERY IN NECROTIZING ENTEROCOLITIS

Necrotizing enterocolitis (NEC) is a devastating disease of prematurity, with no current method with sufficient sensitivity and specificity for early diagnosis. It affects approximately 5% of very low birth weight (VLBW) infants in the United States and is associated with a high mortality rate (20%–30%) and profound morbidity in survivors.[1–3] Diagnosis is particularly challenging, frequently occurring after the disease has progressed to the point of significant and often irreversible intestinal damage. Further complicating clinical management, the disease is typically rapidly progressive, which limits the therapeutic window, resulting in what many experts believe is a

Disclosure Statement: The authors have no commercial or financial conflicts of interest to report.

Funding Sources: G.P. Goldstein received support for the project described in this publication by the Stanford Child Health Research Institute. K.G. Sylvester is supported by NIH 5UL1TR001085-5.

[a] Department of Pediatrics, Stanford University School of Medicine, Palo Alto, CA 94304;
[b] Department of Surgery, Division of Pediatric Surgery, 300 Pasteur Drive, Alway Building M116, MC 5733, Stanford, CA 94305
* Corresponding author. 300 Pasteur Drive, Always Building, M116, MC5733, Stanford, CA 94305.
E-mail address: Sylvester@stanford.edu

predetermined disease course at onset. Despite decades of research, the exact pathophysiology of NEC remains unknown and, accordingly, a clinically useful disease-specific biomarker has not yet been identified. Biomarkers that can either definitively classify the presence of NEC or identify an early, pre-NEC stage of disease are urgently needed.

The critical obstacle to early diagnosis is that the clinical presentation of NEC is nonspecific and varies markedly. When preterm infants develop abdominal distension, emesis, bloody stools, or systemic signs of illness, NEC must be considered in the differential diagnosis. At the onset of symptoms, it is often difficult to precisely make a diagnosis of NEC or differentiate NEC from late-onset sepsis without NEC. Diagnostic uncertainty is more pronounced in the absence of existing clinical confirmatory findings, which has historically involved an abdominal radiograph. Diagnostic criteria include radiographic findings of intestinal perforation (pneumoperitoneum), portal venous gas, or enteric intramural gas (pneumatosis intestinalis), which together or in isolation are considered evidence of significant intestinal injury.[4] Recently, the use of ultrasonography for the detection of abdominal findings that support a diagnosis of NEC, including pneumatosis, suggest that ultrasound as an imaging modality may be more sensitive then plain abdominal radiographs, which can be open to subjective interpretation.[5] Importantly, there has been recent progress in consolidating a working diagnosis of NEC that is clinically contextual and recognizes the developmental window in which NEC most typically occurs, that is, 28 to 32 weeks postmenstrual age.[4]

Given the rapidly progressive nature of the disease, the best strategy to reducing NEC-related mortality and morbidity is prevention of disease onset or its progression. Preventive and treatment measures must be instituted early in disease course. As such, a biomarker identifying NEC at an early stage with ability to monitor disease progression would be highly valuable. Similarly, markers of disease or accurate risk prediction tools would assist in the study of specific intervention designed to prevent or significantly reduce the occurrence of NEC.

Taken together, there are several clinical needs that biomarkers as a class might address when one considers the clinical challenges in managing or preventing NEC: a biomarker would be highly useful in the following clinical scenarios:

1. Risk assessment of likelihood or probability of NEC in all VLBW infants.
2. Early NEC diagnosis, before progression of disease to irreversible intestinal injury.
3. Excluding NEC in infants with symptoms suspicious for NEC (ie, high negative predictive value and specificity).
4. Early NEC prognostication, determining which newborns are likely to have disease progression.

The goal of this review is to discuss the need for novel biomarkers in NEC management, evaluate studies investigating existing biomarkers, and discuss the difficulties associated with translating biomarker discovery into clinical use.

BIOMARKER DEFINITION AND UTILITY

Biomarkers are by definition objective, quantifiable characteristics of biological processes.[6] The National Institutes of Health and Food and Drug Administration produced a document entitled *BEST* (Biomarkers, EndpointS, and other Tools) Resource that provides extensive guidance on the various types and utility of biomarkers, for example, diagnostic, prognostic, predictive, surrogate end-point, etc.[7] BEST defines a biomarker as "a defined characteristic that is measured as an indicator of normal biological processes, pathogenic processes, or response to an exposure or intervention. Molecular, histologic, radiographic, or physiologic characteristics are types of biomarkers." Biomarkers can be used for diagnosis, staging, evaluating response to treatment, predicting response to treatment, and prognostication of outcome. Accordingly, the myriad of studies of molecular biomarkers and radiographic modalities seeking to diagnose and prognose NEC are consistent with the BEST definition of biomarkers.

EVALUATING BIOMARKERS

A biomarker must be measured accurately, reproducibly, and determined to have validity and appropriateness for use. The process of assessing the quality of a biomarker consists of determining if the biomarker has adequate reliability and validity.[8] Reliability refers to the degree to which the results obtained by a measurement procedure can be replicated. The reliability of a biomarker must be established before validity can be assessed. If the biomarker cannot be determined to provide an equivalent result on repeated determinations on the same biological material, it will not be useful for practical application. The validity of a biomarker is defined by the extent to which it measures what it is intended to measure. For example, to establish validity of a biomarker to be used for the diagnosis of NEC, there must be close agreement between the classification of the disease by the biomarker and by the gold standard.

Accuracy of an individual biomarker may be assessed in terms of sensitivity, specificity, area under the receiver operating characteristic (ROC) curve (AUC), positive predictive value (PPV), negative predicative value (NPV), and likelihood ratios (LR).[9,10] Sensitivity and specificity are related to the concept of validity. The sensitivity of a test is its ability to recognize correctly persons who have a condition, that is, the proportion of patients who have a disorder (based on the gold standard) in whom the results of the *test* are positive. The specificity of a test is the ability of a *test* to correctly recognize patients who do not have a condition. It is the proportion of patients who do not have a disorder in whom the test result is negative. PPV is the proportion of patients testing positive who actually have the condition in question. NPV is the proportion of patients testing negative who actually do not have the condition in question. LR is defined as the likelihood that a patient who has a target disorder will have a positive test result, indicated by how much the results of a given diagnostic test result will increase (or decrease) the pretest probability of the target disorder.

Performance of a composite biomarker, such as a prediction model incorporating multiple biomarkers, may be assessed in terms of discrimination and calibration.[11,12] The extent to which the model comes close to achieving the goal of accurately identifying every patient who will develop an event without misclassification can be characterized by the 2 related properties of discrimination and calibration. *Discrimination* is a measure of how well a model distinguishes between 2 outcomes. *Calibration* refers to the agreement between observed outcomes and predicted outcomes.

For binary outcomes (eg, NEC or no NEC), discrimination is typically characterized using ROC curves.[13] After taking all possible pairs of patients and comparing the predicted probabilities, if the model cannot discriminate between patients who will and will NOT have an event, the area under the ROC curve, or c-statistic, is 0.5 (ie, no better than chance). If the model always produces a higher probability for patients having events versus those not having events, the c-statistic is 1.0. The true-positive and false-positive rates must be balanced against each other by choosing a cut-off point or threshold of the test result that maximizes sensitivity and/or specificity. Choosing a cut-off point that increases the true-positive rate will increase the false-positive rate, and in contrast choosing a threshold value with a low rate of true positives will increase the false negatives. The clinical question being considered and the consequences of wrongfully classifying patients should be considered when determining cut-off points for test applications to the target population.

In addition, clinicians need to understand a model's calibration, because a model can have excellent discrimination, but be poorly calibrated and thus provide misleading estimates about absolute risks.[13] Calibration is often considered the most important property of a model and reflects the extent to which a model correctly estimates the absolute risk in the population to which it is applied. Poorly calibrated models will underestimate or overestimate the outcome of interest. A visual representation of the relationship between predicted and observed is the best way to evaluate calibration. An alternative is to evaluate the difference between the predicted and the observed values using statistical tests (eg, the Hosmer-Lemeshow X^2 statistic for goodness-of-fit) to determine whether chance can explain the difference between the predicted and the observed event rate. Above all, measures of biomarker calibration should be reported in a manner that can be clinically interpreted and has relevance to the potential impact of the clinical decision that may follow biomarker utilization.

EVALUATING NECROTIZING ENTEROCOLITIS BIOMARKERS

NEC biomarkers may be developed for the purpose of assisting diagnosis or prognosis. A good biomarker to aid in NEC evaluation requires either high sensitivity or high specificity depending on the clinician's goal. A biomarker to "rule-out" NEC is clinically useful given the uncertainty surrounding initial diagnosis in a patient with nonspecific, but concerning symptoms for NEC. A biomarker for such situation requires high sensitivity and can afford to have moderate specificity. In fact, given the low prevalence of NEC across preterm infant populations, achieving a high sensitivity for such a biomarker will come at the cost of a high false-positive rate, reducing the specificity. Conversely, a biomarker "ruling-in" the disease requires high specificity, high positive predictive value, and a low false-positive rate. To extend the example, the risk of denying treatment must be balanced against the risk of the treatment itself if the test has a low positive predictive value.

ROC curves must be assessed for shape and not merely compared by c-statistic. Given the clinical utility of having an NEC biomarker with either high sensitivity or high specificity, a biomarker study producing a skewed ROC curve is the most pragmatic solution to producing cut-off points that optimize either sensitivity or specificity, because a biomarker with a c-statistic near 1.0 with both optimal sensitivity and specificity is unlikely attainable. **Fig. 1** portrays 2 skewed ROC curves with the ability to select points with emphasis favoring sensitivity or specificity, while demonstrating the effect of choosing on the other metric.

Key challenges for studies evaluating NEC biomarkers include patient selection, study size, and statistical performance. For example, choosing a nonill control group in determining the diagnostic performance of a test for early NEC may lead to exaggerated test performance. In addition, when comparing biomarker classification of NEC to a gold standard definition, broadly considered as surgical findings of intestinal inflammation or necrosis or imaging findings of pneumatosis or pneumoperitoneum, one must consider that the gold standard is specific to highly progressed disease but insensitive to early disease. Therefore, biomarker studies that seek to identify early NEC must not use surgical NEC because this limits the ability to adequately assess for

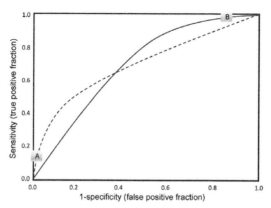

Fig. 1. Hypothetical receiving operating curves of biomarkers for NEC diagnosis. Two hypothetical curves are shown representing the discriminatory capacity of 2 models. The ROC curves depict performance of potentially useful biomarkers for NEC diagnosis. Each model correctly classifies more patients with events than misclassifies patients without events (AUC ~ 0.7). Point A shows a cut-off that has high specificity, but low sensitivity. Point B shows a test with high sensitivity and low specificity.

early, nonprogressive, (ie, medical) NEC. A pragmatic approach for a gold-standard diagnostic criteria for early, nonprogressive NEC is also uncertain and has hampered many efforts to date in biomarkers discovery work. Furthermore, biomarker studies of NEC should restrict the study patient population to NEC in preterm infants. Historically, clinicians have associated several diseases together under the umbrella of NEC, including spontaneous intestinal perforation and intestinal necrosis in full-term infants. However, the belief that preterm NEC is likely a distinct disease suggests that diagnosis should be reserved for those newborns who meet appropriate preterm gestational age and postmenstrual age correction criteria. The common misconception that pneumatosis and pneumoperitoneum are pathognomonic of NEC, irrespective of gestational and developmental age, has resulted in a variety of other gastrointestinal pathologies being possibly falsely labeled NEC including full-term infants with congenital heart disease resulting from poor perfusion to the intestine and food protein–induced enterocolitis syndrome (FPIES).[4] Thus biomarker studies that fail to separate these distinct groups when assessing clinical validity invoke misclassification bias. A recent article by Gephart and colleagues[4] discusses the challenges surrounding the creation of a precise definition for NEC and describes a 2 out of 3 rule for NEC diagnosis based on expert opinion from the 2017 NEC symposium. Finally, control group selection has important ramifications on interpretation of results. For example, a biomarker with good specificity for NEC must be assessed in comparison with patients with late-onset sepsis without NEC, given the large overlap in clinical symptoms between these groups.

NECROTIZING ENTEROCOLITIS PATHOPHYSIOLOGY

NEC biomarker research should focus on markers that are consistent with or describe a relevant biological perspective of NEC pathophysiology. From a biological perspective, the ideal NEC biomarker would correspond to a proximal component of the pathophysiologic cascade. A key challenge in NEC biomarker discovery is that we currently have an incomplete understanding of its pathophysiology.

Regardless, rigorous biomarker research is likely to advance our understanding of NEC.

See **Table 1** for summary of notable biomarkers studied for NEC diagnosis or prognostication. Of note, biomarker studies without clinical data (ie, only preclinical) were not included.

Abdominal Ultrasound

Janssen Lok and colleagues[5] performed a systematic review of 15 studies assessing abdominal ultrasound for diagnosis of NEC. The investigators reported substantial heterogeneity among the studies, most with low sensitivities (<70%) and some with fair specificities (>80%) for NEC. They concluded that for abdominal ultrasound to add value to management of NEC, a well-designed prospective study is needed in diagnosing NEC and its progression.

Calprotectin

Calprotectin from stool is a plausible choice of a biomarker for NEC given its utility in patients with inflammatory bowel disease. It belongs to a family of calcium-binding proteins that are expressed in phagocytes, monocytes, macrophages, and granulocytes. Calprotectin proteins are released into the gastrointestinal tract during intestinal inflammation, resulting from increased neutrophil migration toward the intestinal mucosa. MacQueen and colleagues[14] assessed fecal calprotectin in 118 preterm infants undergoing evaluation for NEC, of which 33 were eventually diagnosed with it. They reported that a stool calprotectin level of 299 µg/g was the value with the best cutoff point, having a sensitivity of 71% and specificity of 88%. In addition, Pergialiotis and colleagues[15] performed a systematic review of calprotectin levels in NEC, assessing 13 studies, involving 601 patients. They found wide variations in sensitivities (76%–100%) and specificities (39%–96%), AUCs (0.65–0.89), and calprotectin cut-off points (280–792 µg/g).

Claudins

Claudins are tight junction proteins expressed in high quantity in the intestine and have potential biomarker utility given the loss of intestinal wall integrity in the setting of NEC. Thuijls and colleagues[16] assessed 35 infants with suspicion for NEC, of which 14 were ultimately diagnosed with it. Median urinary claudin-3 levels were significantly higher in neonates with NEC. The investigators reported a cut-off point of 801 INT with sensitivity of 71%, specificity of 81%, and AUC of 0.76 to diagnose NEC Bell stage greater than or equal to 2.

Complete Blood Cell Count

Hematological indices such as total white blood cell (WBC) count, absolute neutrophil count, percent bandemia, immature to total white blood cell ratio (I:T ratio), and platelet count are commonly used in the evaluation of suspected NEC. Gordon and colleagues[17] assessed 5166 infants with NEC, 1107 of whom died, and evaluated complete blood count characteristics at NEC diagnosis associated with mortality. They found that a high total WBC, elevated I:T ratio, low platelet count, and high absolute monocyte count were associated with increased mortality. In addition, thrombocytopenia is seen at clinical presentation of NEC in 50% to 95% of cases and most neonates with advanced NEC develop thrombocytopenia within 24 to 72 hours of onset of disease.[18] Moreover, the severity of thrombocytopenia correlates with the Bell's clinical stage of NEC.[19]

Table 1
Assessment of biomarkers evaluated for necrotizing enterocolitis diagnosis

Biomarkers	Sample Source	Sensitivity[a]	Specificity[a]	Strengths (S) and Limitations (L)	References
Abdominal ultrasound	Ultrasound	Low	Low to high	L: high specificity may be limited to more advanced disease L: low sensitivity	Janssen Lok et al,[5] 2018
Calprotectin	Stool	Low-high	Low-medium	S: levels are usually elevated in patients with NEC and correlate with disease severity. L: can be elevated in preterm infants for reasons besides NEC, limiting its specificity. L: sensitivity not consistently high across studies to warrant use as a biomarker to accurately "rule-out" NEC.	MacQueen et al,[14] 2016 Pergialiotis et al,[15] 2016
CBC	Serum			L: elements of CBC are not sensitive or specific for NEC.	Gordon et al,[17] 2016
Claudins	Urine	Low	Low	L: associated with NEC, but sensitivity and specificity are low.	Thuijs et al,[16] 2010
CRP	Serum	Low-High	Low	S: unlikely normal in the setting of NEC, although sensitivities among studies varies. L: relatively slow increase, rendering it impractical for early diagnosis. L: low specificity.	Cetinkaya et al,[44] 2011 Pourcyrous et al,[25] 2005 Yakut et al,[36] 2014
Cytokines	Serum			S: IL-6, IL-8, and IL-10 are associated with NEC, and IL-8 seems to have high sensitivity and specificity. L: IL-8 has only been studied to a limited extent.	Benkoe et al,[22] 2013 Benkoe et al,[23] 2014
C5a	Serum			L: strongly associated with NEC although has only been studied to a limited extent.	Tayman et al,[21] 2011
EGF	Serum			L: limited investigation. No reported validity testing.	Shin et al,[27] 2000 Nair et al,[26] 2008

(continued on next page)

Table 1
(continued)

Biomarkers	Sample Source	Sensitivity[a]	Specificity[a]	Strengths (S) and Limitations (L)	References
Genomics	Serum			S: variants found to be associated with NEC. L: no studies assess accuracy of variants in NEC diagnosis or prognostication. L: expensive.	Sampath et al,[28] 2017 Härtel et al,[29] 2016 Chan et al,[30] 2014 Treszl et al,[31] 2003 Prencipe et al,[32] 2012
Hydrogen extraction	Exhaled breath	Medium	Medium	S: noninvasive collection and moderate sensitivity and specificity. L: limited investigation.	Cheu et al,[33] 1989
I-FABP	Serum or urine	Low	Medium	S: moderate specificity (91%) for serum I-FABP in meta-analysis of 7 studies. L: low sensitivity and specificity for urinary I-FABP.	Yang et al,[35] 2016
IAIP	Serum	High	Medium	S: high sensitivity and NPV. May be very useful for ruling out NEC in suspected cases. L: limited investigation. L: unclear whether Iaip can distinguish NEC from sepsis.	Shah et al,[34] 2017
Metabolomics	Serum or urine			S: population-based assessment of metabolic screen utility for identifying high risk of NEC (Sylvester). S: metabolites linked to possible NEC-linked dysbiosis (Morrow). L: poor PPV	Morrow et al,[39] 2013 Sylvester et al,[38] 2017
IMA	Serum	Medium	Low	S: high sensitivity than CRP in one study. L: limited investigation.	Yakut et al,[36] 2014

Biomarker	Source					References
Microbiota analysis	Stool	Low-High	Low-High	Low-High	S: very high sensitivity and specificity with different models reported in one study. L: inconsistency in microbiome profiles across studies. L: limited sample size for models with high sensitivity and specificity.	Morrow et al,[39] 2013 Pammi et al,[40] 2017
NIRS	Skin lead				S: possible use for monitoring course after initial NEC diagnosis to detect complications.	Shah et al,[34] 2017
PAF	Serum and Stool				S: associated with NEC. L: low specificity. L: limited investigation.	Amer et al,[42] 2014
Procalcitonin	Serum	Low-Medium	High		S: high specificity if limited to patients with NEC and sepsis. L: unable to identify patients with NEC without sepsis.	Cetinkaya et al,[44] 2011 Turner et al,[43] 2007
Proteomics	Serum or urine	Medium	Low		S: moderate sensitivity in panel of 7 urinary proteins. L: limited evaluation	Sylvester et al,[47] 2014
SAA	Serum or urine	Low	Low		L: low sensitivity and specificity.	Cetinkaya et al,[48] 2010 Reisinger et al,[49] 2014
S100A12	Stool	Low	Low		L: associated with NEC, but low sensitivity and specificity.	Däbritz et al,[50] 2012
TFF3	Serum	Low	High		S: high specificity for very elevated values. L: low sensitivity. L: limited investigation.	Ng et al[37]
VOCs	Stool	Medium	Medium		S: noninvasive collection and moderate sensitivity and specificity. S: discriminates NEC well from patients with sepsis. L: limited investigation.	de Meij et al,[51] 2015

Abbreviations: IMA, ischemia-modified albumin; ITF, intestinal trefoil factor; NIRS, near-infrared spectroscopy; PAF, platelet-activating factor; SAA, serum amyloid-A protein; TFF, trefoil factor; VOC, volatile organic compound.

[a] High: greater than 95%; Medium: 85% to 95%; Low: less than 85%.

Compliment Component 5a

C5a is a potent proinflammatory mediator cleaved enzymatically from its precursor, C5, on activation of the complement cascade.[20] Tayman and colleagues[21] assessed 22 preterm infants with NEC and 23 matched controls. The investigators found that serum levels of C5a were significantly higher in infants with NEC. They also found that an AUC for C5a (0.83, 0.88) was significantly higher than for C-reactive protein (CRP) (0.69, 0.69) and interleukin 6 (IL-6) (0.66, 0.71) at the time of NEC diagnosis for predicting need for surgery and mortality.

Cytokines

Cytokines are proteins that regulate the immune response and can be released during early phases of the innate immune response, making them an attractive target for early identification of NEC. Benkoe and colleagues[22] assessed a battery of 11 cytokines, including IL-12, IFN-c, IL-2, IL-10, IL-8, IL-6, IL-4, IL-5, IL-1b, tumor necrosis factor alpha (TNF-a), and TNF-b, in 9 infants with NEC and 18 matched controls. The investigators reported that only 3 cytokines, IL-6, IL-8, and IL-10, were significantly associated with surgical NEC. Benkoe and colleagues[23] assessed 15 infants with NEC and 14 matched controls and reported an AUC of 0.99.

C-Reactive Protein

CRP is produced in the liver and increases in the serum in response to inflammation. In acute inflammation, CRP can increase within 4 to 6 hours, doubles every 8 hours, and reaches its peak at 36 to 50 hours following injury or inflammation. Its half-life is about 19 hours.[24] The delayed and relatively slow increase in CRP renders it impractical for use because many cases of NEC progress faster than the time CRP will increase. Pourcyrous and colleagues[25] demonstrated the utility of using CRP in the setting of patients with gastrointestinal (GI) symptoms to discriminate benign GI symptoms from NEC. A normal CRP was seen in 1 out of 66 patients with NEC, indicating its high, although not perfect, sensitivity to rule out advanced NEC. Alternatively, elevated CRP levels were not specific to NEC and were seen in patients found to have a variety of other disorders, including urinary tract infection, pneumonia, meningitis, bacteremia, sepsis of unclear cause, meconium aspiration syndrome, and maternal disorders.

Epidermal Growth Factor

Growth factors play an important role in GI tract development.[26] Shin and colleagues[27] found that epidermal growth factor levels were significantly lower in saliva and in the serum in patients with NEC compared with control patients, whereas urinary levels were not significantly different.

Genomics

Genomics involves sequencing and analysis of DNA and genes. The genetic basis of NEC remains unknown, although is increasingly being scrutinized. Several studies have assessed specific genes in patients with NEC versus controls and identified variants associated with NEC.[28–32] NEC pathophysiology does not seem to be explained by a single gene. Gene testing may be helpful in NEC prognostication. To our knowledge, biomarker validity testing has not been performed with these variants to evaluate accuracy of a genomic biomarker (single or panel) for NEC diagnosis or prognostication.

Hydrogen Excretion

Breath hydrogen excretion has been used to diagnose malabsorption and bacterial overgrowth syndromes given that intestinal bacteria produce hydrogen by fermentation of unabsorbed carbohydrates. Cheu and colleagues[33] assessed breath hydrogen excretion in 122 neonates and found that a value of greater than or equal to 8.0 ppm/mm Hg resulted in a sensitivity of 86% and a specificity of 90% for NEC diagnosis.

Inter-Alpha Inhibitor Protein

IAIP is a serine protease inhibitor that helps regulate inflammation and is a negative acute-phase reactant. Shah and colleagues[34] assessed 14 preterm infants with NEC, 13 with SIP, and 26 matched controls. They found that mean IAIP levels were significantly lower in the NEC group. ROC analysis for NEC yielded an AUC of 0.98, a sensitivity of 100%, a specificity of 88%, a PPV of 41%, and an NPV of 100%.

Intestinal Fatty Acid-Binding Protein

Intestinal fatty acid-binding protein (I-FABP) is a cytoplasmic protein expressed in high quantities in enterocytes and is released into circulation on intestinal cell wall injury. In a recent systematic review, Yang and colleagues[35] assessed I-FABP for diagnosis of NEC in 14 studies. They reported pooled serum I-FABP performance statistics: sensitivity 64%, specificity 91%, and AUC 0.84. Urinary I-FABP sensitivity was similar to serum sensitivity but specificity was lower (73%).

Ischemia-Modified Albumin

Ischemia-modified albumin (IMA) increases in the blood after an ischemic event. Yakut and colleagues[36] assessed 37 preterm infants with NEC and 36 matched controls. IMA was significantly increased in patients with NEC compared with controls. At time of NEC diagnosis, IMA sensitivity was 89%, specificity was 64%, and AUC was 0.82.

Intestinal Trefoil Factors

Trefoil factors (TFF) are secreted by mucin-producing epithelial cells and play an important role in enteral self-protection and repair. Ng and colleagues[37] evaluated TFF3 in 20 preterm infants with NEC, 40 preterm infants with sepsis, and 40 matched controls. They demonstrated a sensitivity of 50% and a specificity of 98% for distinguishing NEC from sepsis and controls.

Metabolomics

Metabolomics is the profiling of small molecule metabolites. Sylvester and colleagues[38] repurposed the newborn screen metabolic data and identified 14 acylcarnitine levels and ratios from newborn blood that were associated with an increased risk of NEC. They created a model that predicted NEC diagnosis with an AUC of 0.90. Similarly, Morrow and colleagues[39] assessed the urinary alanine to histidine ratio and reported a sensitivity of 82% and a specificity of 75% for NEC diagnosis.

Microbiota Analysis

Intestinal dysbiosis is thought to play a central role in NEC pathogenesis. Morrow and colleagues[39] assessed stool samples of preterm infants on day of life 4 to 9 in 11 infants who developed NEC and 21 matched controls. The investigators found that they could develop microbiota models that identified NEC with 100% specificity (ie, high Firmicutes relative abundance) or 100% sensitivity (involving Propionibacterium, Firmicutes dysbiosis, and Proteobacteria dysbiosis). Pammi and colleagues[40] performed a systematic review of 14 studies assessing intestinal dysbiosis in preterm infants preceding NEC. They concluded that there exists inconsistency in the microbiome profiles in stool samples preceding NEC across studies and this may be due to considerable clinical and methodological heterogeneity. They found that intestinal dysbiosis preceding NEC is characterized by increased relative abundances of Proteobacteria and decreased relative abundances of Firmicutes and Bacteroidetes.

Near-Infrared Spectroscopy

Near-infrared spectroscopy (NIRS) is a noninvasive measure of regional tissue oxygenation and has the potential to identify intestinal tissue with poor perfusion. Shah and colleagues[34] assessed intestinal NIRS in 33 patients with suspected NEC, 20 of which developed it. They did not generate ROC curves for intestinal NIRS, although they reported that a liver NIRS threshold of less than 59% has high sensitivity and specificity to differentiate complicated from uncomplicated NEC.

Platelet-Activating Factor

Platelet-activating factor (PAF) is a phospholipid produced by platelets, leukocytes, and endothelial cells during inflammatory responses and is thought to play a central role in NEC pathogenesis.[41] Rabinowitz and colleagues found that serum PAF levels were elevated in NEC cases compared with controls and were associated with disease severity. Amer and colleagues[42] demonstrated that fecal PAF levels are also elevated in cases of NEC compared with controls.

Procalcitonin

Procalcitonin (PCT) is a prohormone of calcitonin that is released from both thyroid and immune cell lines, rising in response to proinflammatory stimuli, especially of bacterial origin. Levels may be increased within 2 to 3 hours in response to invasive infection. Turner and colleagues[43] reported that PCT levels were not elevated in patients with NEC, rather were similar to healthy controls. However, PCT levels were elevated in patients with sepsis. Cetinkaya and colleagues[44] reported a relatively high sensitivity (92%) and specificity (98%) for elevated PCT in patients with NEC and sepsis.

Proteomics

Proteomics is the study of proteins and their interactions and modifications. Several studies have assessed proteomics in patients with NEC or early NEC diagnosis.[45–47] Sylvester and colleagues[47] evaluated a panel of urinary protein biomarkers and reported promising results with differentiating NEC from sepsis, with AUC of 0.98, sensitivity of 89%, and specificity of 80%.

Serum Amyloid-A Protein

Serum amyloid-A protein (SAA) is an apolipoprotein secreted from hepatocytes, endothelial cells, monocytes, and smooth muscle cells and may play a role in regulating inflammation. Mean serum SAA is increased in preterm infants with NEC as compared with those with sepsis alone.[48] Reisinger and colleagues[49] reported that urinary SAA levels were significantly higher in severe NEC, with a sensitivity and a specificity of 83%.

S100A12

S100A12 is a cytosolic calcium-binding protein released by phagocytes on activation during intestinal inflammation. S100A12 may play an important role in innate immunity. Däbritz and colleagues[50] demonstrated that fecal S100A12 levels were greater in preterm infants with NEC compared with controls. With a cut-off value of greater than 210 mg/kg at the time of NEC diagnosis, specificity was 67%, specificity was 78%, and AUC was 0.7.

Volatile Organic Compound Analysis

Fecal volatile organic compounds (VOCs) are carbon-based gaseous chemicals, originating from fermentation of intestinal bacteria of nutrients. de Meij and colleagues[51] assessed fecal VOCs in 13 preterm infants with NEC, 31 with sepsis, and 14 matched controls. They found that VOC profiles assessed 1 day before NEC diagnosis had a sensitivity of 89%, a specificity of 89%, and an AUC of 0.99 for NEC diagnosis. Furthermore, VOC profiles were significantly different in patients with NEC compared with those in patients with sepsis alone.

COMPOSITE BIOMARKERS

An approach to increase biomarker predictive capabilities is to combine multiple biomarkers with readily available clinical markers. This has the potential advantage of quantifying the pretest risk of disease with the observed incidence of disease (ie, discrimination). This type of approach was taken by Sylvester and colleagues in their report of a refined panel of urinary protein biomarkers as having low sensitivity and specificity, but when combined in a panel with clinical parameters provided much greater diagnostic and prognostic accuracy for NEC diagnosis. The development of composite models that use available clinical features together with existing or novel molecular indicators is a pragmatic approach to improving sensitivity and specificity. Multivariate models with standard measures along with Bayesian models that provide conditional probabilities may together provide key differential insights.

SUMMARY

Several biomarker studies report good sensitivities or specificities for NEC diagnosis or prognostication of disease progression. Some of the biomarkers with reported high specificities, however, have not been rigorously assessed in appropriate populations and most do not rigorously report metrics of probability or population calibration. For example, elevated CRP and procalcitonin have been reported to be highly specific for NEC diagnosis in some studies, although these studies do not include a control group of patients with sepsis alone without NEC, leading to misclassification bias. Several biomarkers that report high sensitivities for NEC diagnosis, such as IAIP, hydrogen excretion, VOCs, fecal microbiota analysis, and proteomics, are limited in clinical use given that they have not yet undergone sufficient validity testing with reproduced results. These limitations together with a general absence of prospective validation in multicenter studies to assess analytical validity (reproducibility), clinical validity (discrimination and calibration), and generalizability render most NEC biomarkers published to date of limited clinical utility.

Biomarker research has tremendous potential to advance clinical management of NEC and our understanding of its pathogenesis. A variety of biomarkers have been shown to perform with good sensitivity or specificity for NEC diagnosis, such as IAIP, hydrogen excretion, VOCs, fecal microbiota, analysis, and proteomics, but each of these require further validity testing. Overall, there is a need for multicenter validation studies of already existing NEC biomarkers. This may be facilitated by a multi-center biorepository that is being developed by the NEC Society. Furthermore, future biomarker literature must report on reliability and validity as well as appropriate performance parameters such as sensitivity, specificity, PPV, NPV, LRs, AUC, discrimination, and calibration. To enhance performance, utilization of a composite biomarker with multiple high-performing parameters is more likely to provide meaningful advancement to the field than single biomarkers. Biomarker studies must use appropriate study populations given the intended goal of the biomarker, because studies are prone to misclassification bias. Finally, in the authors' opinion, the greatest unmet need in NEC biomarker discovery is the lack of an early disease marker for NEC. Identifying a sensitive and specific biomarker that diagnoses NEC at a preclinical gut injury stage would be revolutionary to the field and pave the way for substantial reduction in NEC related mortality and morbidity.

Best practices

What is the current practice for Necrotizing Enterocolitis?

A. Necrotizing Enterocolitis (NEC), a devastating acquired disease of the gastro-intestinal tract that exclusively affects premature neonates. There are currently no approved or validated blood tests or biomarkers that are diagnostic of NEC. The lack of validated biomarkers has hindered population based reporting and clinical trials for NEC.

What changes in current practice are likely to improve outcomes?

A. The development of biomarkers for NEC has the potential to advance clinical management and deepen the understanding of its pathophysiology.

Is there a clinical algorithm?

A. This review summarizes some of the relevant performance metrics like discrimination and calibration, that are required to develop and validate an effective biomarker of NEC.

Major Recommendations

A. This review provides an analysis of candidate biomarkers of NEC and their reported performance metrics. Recommendations for the much-needed prospective validation of NEC biomarkers are discussed.

Strength of the Evidence?

A. Highly variable depending on the candidate biomarker under consideration, **Table 1**.

Current Sources.

A. All utilized and relevant sources appear indexed in PubMed.

Summary Statement.

Biomarker research has tremendous potential to advance clinical management of NEC and deepen an understanding of its pathogenesis. A variety of biomarkers have been shown to perform with good sensitivity or specificity for NEC diagnosis, but each of these require further validity testing. Identifying a sensitive and relatively specific biomarker that diagnoses NEC at a pre-clinical gut injury stage would be revolutionary to the field and pave the way for substantial reduction in NEC related mortality and morbidity.

REFERENCES

1. Horbar JD, Edwards EM, Greenberg LT, et al. Variation in performance of neonatal intensive care units in the United States. JAMA Pediatr 2017;171(3): e164396.
2. Stoll BJ, Hansen NI, Bell EF, et al. Trends in care practices, morbidity, and mortality of extremely preterm neonates, 1993-2012. JAMA 2015;314(10): 1039–51.
3. Neu J, Walker WA. Necrotizing enterocolitis. N Engl J Med 2011;364(3):255–64.

4. Gephart SM, Gordon PV, Penn AH, et al. Changing the paradigm of defining, detecting, and diagnosing NEC: perspectives on Bell's stages and biomarkers for NEC. Semin Pediatr Surg 2018;27(1):3–10.

5. Janssen Lok M, Miyake H, Hock A, et al. Value of abdominal ultrasound in management of necrotizing enterocolitis: a systematic review and meta-analysis. Pediatr Surg Int 2018. https://doi.org/10.1007/s00383-018-4259-8.

6. Strimbu K, Tavel JA. What are biomarkers? Curr Opin HIV AIDS 2010;5(6):463–6.

7. BEST (Biomarkers, EndpointS, and other Tools) Resource - PubMed - NCBI. Available at: https://www-ncbi-nlm-nih-gov.laneproxy.stanford.edu/pubmed/27010052. Accessed May 19, 2018.

8. Looney SW. Statistical methods for assessing biomarkers. Methods Mol Biol 2002;184:81–109.

9. Eusebi P. Diagnostic accuracy measures. Cerebrovasc Dis 2013;36(4):267–72.

10. Taylor JMG, Ankerst DP, Andridge RR. Validation of biomarker-based risk prediction models. Clin Cancer Res 2008;14(19):5977–83.

11. Moons KGM, Altman DG, Reitsma JB, et al. Transparent reporting of a multivariable prediction model for individual prognosis or diagnosis (TRIPOD): explanation and elaboration. Ann Intern Med 2015;162(1):W1–73.

12. Collins GS, Reitsma JB, Altman DG, et al. Transparent reporting of a multivariable prediction model for individual prognosis or diagnosis (TRIPOD): the TRIPOD statement. Br J Surg 2015;102(3):148–58.

13. Alba AC, Agoritsas T, Walsh M, et al. Discrimination and calibration of clinical prediction models: users' guides to the medical literature. JAMA 2017;318(14):1377–84.

14. MacQueen BC, Christensen RD, Yost CC, et al. Elevated fecal calprotectin levels during necrotizing enterocolitis are associated with activated neutrophils extruding neutrophil extracellular traps. J Perinatol 2016;36(10):862–9.

15. Pergialiotis V, Konstantopoulos P, Karampetsou N, et al. Calprotectin levels in necrotizing enterocolitis: a systematic review of the literature. Inflamm Res 2016;65(11):847–52.

16. Thuijls G, Derikx JPM, van Wijck K, et al. Non-invasive markers for early diagnosis and determination of the severity of necrotizing enterocolitis. Ann Surg 2010;251(6):1174–80.

17. Gordon PV, Swanson JR, Clark R, et al. The complete blood cell count in a refined cohort of preterm NEC: the importance of gestational age and day of diagnosis when using the CBC to estimate mortality. J Perinatol 2016;36(2):121–5.

18. Maheshwari A. Immunologic and hematological abnormalities in necrotizing enterocolitis. Clin Perinatol 2015;42(3):567–85.

19. Ververidis M, Kiely EM, Spitz L, et al. The clinical significance of thrombocytopenia in neonates with necrotizing enterocolitis. J Pediatr Surg 2001;36(5):799–803.

20. Manthey HD, Woodruff TM, Taylor SM, et al. Complement component 5a (C5a). Int J Biochem Cell Biol 2009;41(11):2114–7.

21. Tayman C, Tonbul A, Kahveci H, et al. C5a, a complement activation product, is a useful marker in predicting the severity of necrotizing enterocolitis. Tohoku J Exp Med 2011;224(2):143–50.

22. Benkoe T, Baumann S, Weninger M, et al. Comprehensive evaluation of 11 cytokines in premature infants with surgical necrotizing enterocolitis. PLoS One 2013;8(3):e58720.

23. Benkoe TM, Mechtler TP, Weninger M, et al. Serum levels of interleukin-8 and gut-associated biomarkers in diagnosing necrotizing enterocolitis in preterm infants. J Pediatr Surg 2014;49(10):1446–51.

24. Litao MKS, Kamat D. Erythrocyte sedimentation rate and C-reactive protein: how best to use them in clinical practice. Pediatr Ann 2014;43(10):417–20.

25. Pourcyrous M, Korones SB, Yang W, et al. C-reactive protein in the diagnosis, management, and prognosis of neonatal necrotizing enterocolitis. Pediatrics 2005;116(5):1064–9.

26. Nair RR, Warner BB, Warner BW. Role of epidermal growth factor and other growth factors in the prevention of necrotizing enterocolitis. Semin Perinatol 2008;32(2):107–13.

27. Shin CE, Falcone RA, Stuart L, et al. Diminished epidermal growth factor levels in infants with necrotizing enterocolitis. J Pediatr Surg 2000;35(2):173–6 [discussion: 177].

28. Sampath V, Bhandari V, Berger J, et al. A functional ATG16L1 (T300A) variant is associated with necrotizing enterocolitis in premature infants. Pediatr Res 2017; 81(4):582–8.

29. Härtel C, Hartz A, Pagel J, et al. NOD2 loss-of-function mutations and risks of necrotizing enterocolitis or focal intestinal perforation in very low-birth-weight infants. Inflamm Bowel Dis 2016;22(2):249–56.

30. Chan KYY, Leung KT, Tam YH, et al. Genome-wide expression profiles of necrotizing enterocolitis versus spontaneous intestinal perforation in human intestinal tissues: dysregulation of functional pathways. Ann Surg 2014;260(6):1128–37.

31. Treszl A, Héninger E, Kálmán A, et al. Lower prevalence of IL-4 receptor alpha-chain gene G variant in very-low-birth-weight infants with necrotizing enterocolitis. J Pediatr Surg 2003;38(9):1374–8.

32. Prencipe G, Azzari C, Moriondo M, et al. Association between mannose-binding lectin gene polymorphisms and necrotizing enterocolitis in preterm infants. J Pediatr Gastroenterol Nutr 2012;55(2):160–5.

33. Cheu HW, Brown DR, Rowe MI. Breath hydrogen excretion as a screening test for the early diagnosis of necrotizing enterocolitis. Am J Dis Child 1989;143(2): 156–9.

34. Shah BA, Migliori A, Kurihara I, et al. Blood level of inter-alpha inhibitor proteins distinguishes necrotizing enterocolitis from spontaneous intestinal perforation. J Pediatr 2017;180:135–40.e1.

35. Yang G, Wang Y, Jiang X. Diagnostic value of intestinal fatty-acid-binding protein in necrotizing enterocolitis: a systematic review and meta-analysis. Indian J Pediatr 2016;83(12–13):1410–9.

36. Yakut I, Tayman C, Oztekin O, et al. Ischemia-modified albumin may be a novel marker for the diagnosis and follow-up of necrotizing enterocolitis. J Clin Lab Anal 2014;28(3):170–7.

37. Ng EWY, Poon TCW, Lam HS, et al. Gut-associated biomarkers L-FABP, I-FABP, and TFF3 and LIT score for diagnosis of surgical necrotizing enterocolitis in preterm infants. Ann Surg 2013;258(6):1111–8.

38. Sylvester KG, Kastenberg ZJ, Moss RL, et al. Acylcarnitine profiles reflect metabolic vulnerability for necrotizing enterocolitis in newborns born premature. J Pediatr 2017;181:80–5.e1.

39. Morrow AL, Lagomarcino AJ, Schibler KR, et al. Early microbial and metabolomic signatures predict later onset of necrotizing enterocolitis in preterm infants. Microbiome 2013;1(1):13.

40. Pammi M, Cope J, Tarr PI, et al. Intestinal dysbiosis in preterm infants preceding necrotizing enterocolitis: a systematic review and meta-analysis. Microbiome 2017;5(1):31.
41. Frost BL, Caplan MS. Necrotizing enterocolitis: pathophysiology, platelet-activating factor, and probiotics. Semin Pediatr Surg 2013;22(2):88–93.
42. Amer MD, Hedlund E, Rochester J, et al. Platelet-activating factor concentration in the stool of human newborns: effects of enteral feeding and neonatal necrotizing enterocolitis. Biol Neonate 2004;85(3):159–66.
43. Turner D, Hammerman C, Rudensky B, et al. Low levels of procalcitonin during episodes of necrotizing enterocolitis. Dig Dis Sci 2007;52(11):2972–6.
44. Cetinkaya M, Ozkan H, Köksal N, et al. Comparison of the efficacy of serum amyloid A, C-reactive protein, and procalcitonin in the diagnosis and follow-up of necrotizing enterocolitis in premature infants. J Pediatr Surg 2011;46(8):1482–9.
45. Jiang P, Smith B, Qvist N, et al. Intestinal proteome changes during infant necrotizing enterocolitis. Pediatr Res 2013;73(3):268–76.
46. Ng PC, Ang IL, Chiu RWK, et al. Host-response biomarkers for diagnosis of late-onset septicemia and necrotizing enterocolitis in preterm infants. J Clin Invest 2010;120(8):2989–3000.
47. Sylvester KG, Ling XB, Liu GY-G, et al. Urine protein biomarkers for the diagnosis and prognosis of necrotizing enterocolitis in infants. J Pediatr 2014;164(3):607–12.e1-7.
48. Cetinkaya M, Ozkan H, Köksal N, et al. The efficacy of serial serum amyloid A measurements for diagnosis and follow-up of necrotizing enterocolitis in premature infants. Pediatr Surg Int 2010;26(8):835–41.
49. Reisinger KW, Kramer BW, Van der Zee DC, et al. Non-invasive serum amyloid A (SAA) measurement and plasma platelets for accurate prediction of surgical intervention in severe necrotizing enterocolitis (NEC). PLoS One 2014;9(6):e90834.
50. Däbritz J, Jenke A, Wirth S, et al. Fecal phagocyte-specific S100A12 for diagnosing necrotizing enterocolitis. J Pediatr 2012;161(6):1059–64.
51. de Meij TGJ, van der Schee MPC, Berkhout DJC, et al. Early detection of necrotizing enterocolitis by fecal volatile organic compounds analysis. J Pediatr 2015;167(3):562–7.e1.

Challenges in Advancing Necrotizing Enterocolitis Research

Cheryl Battersby, MBChB, FRCPCH, PhD,
Neena Modi, MBChB, FRCP, FRCPCH, MD*

KEYWORDS

* Necrotizing enterocolitis * Preclinical research * Clinical trials

KEY POINTS

* Progressing necrotizing enterocolitis (NEC) research is difficult because the disease is variable in presentation, there are difficulties in making a precise diagnosis, a reliable agreed case-definition is currently lacking, and there is a paucity of preclinical research to identify etiologic targets.
* The major challenges of the cost of clinical trials and need for long-term outcome ascertainment could be eased through incorporation of novel randomization approaches and data collection into routine care, and collaboration between public-sector and industry funders.
* The rarity of severe NEC calls for collaboration across national and international boundaries to deliver studies with adequate power to address important outcomes and identify and test candidate biomarkers of disease risk, diagnosis and prognosis.
* There is need to engage with regulators, and with parents and the public, to widen perspectives when evaluating the safety and effectiveness of potential therapies for NEC.

BACKGROUND

Necrotizing enterocolitis (NEC) is an enigmatic disease. Parents and clinicians alike fear NEC because it can strike devastatingly, and without warning. It is primarily, but not exclusively, a disease that affects extremely preterm infants, and thus, as survival of the most immature has increased, so too has the incidence of NEC. High-income countries now rank NEC among the leading causes of mortality and long-term morbidity in the extremely preterm population, and the need to improve prevention and treatment of this disease is clear. Here, the authors discuss the many challenges in advancing NEC research and offer suggestions for a way forward.

Section of Neonatal Medicine, Department of Medicine, Chelsea and Westminster Hospital campus, 369 Fulham Road, London SW10 9NH
* Corresponding author.
E-mail address: n.modi@imperial.ac.uk

Clin Perinatol 46 (2019) 19–27
https://doi.org/10.1016/j.clp.2018.10.002
0095-5108/19/© 2018 Elsevier Inc. All rights reserved.

DEFINING THE DISEASE

NEC is protean in its presentation. Severe disease characteristically presents clinically with features of an ileus (abdominal distension, bilious aspirates/vomiting), intestinal inflammation (abdominal tenderness), and intestinal necrosis (bloody stools, bowel perforation). There may be signs of systemic sepsis (poor peripheral perfusion, hypotension, shock, multiorgan dysfunction). Radiographical features (fixed dilated bowel loops, bowel wall thickening, pneumatosis, portal venous gas, pneumoperitoneum) mirror clinical findings, as do laboratory parameters (increase in acute phase reactants, positive blood cultures, coagulopathy). At the other end of the spectrum, the onset of NEC may be marked by no more than enteral intolerance with mild abdominal distension, and other nonspecific features, commonplace in neonatal intensive care unit populations. There are no definitive diagnostic tests, and therefore, because of the fear in which the disease is held, clinical practice is cautious, leading to frequent episodes of withholding enteral feeds for varying periods of time that in itself may paradoxically increase the risk of NEC because enteral substrate promotes intestinal growth and integrity. Clinical assessment is largely subjective; hence ascertainment bias is a major possibility in unblinded clinical trials. To further complicate matters, it is also unclear if NEC is a single entity because several other gastrointestinal pathologic conditions share clinical, radiological, and laboratory parameters in common such as spontaneous intestinal perforation (SIP), cytomegalovirus enteritis, and intestinal dysmotility syndromes.

CASE DEFINITION

Although clearly of great importance for case ascertainment, there is no internationally agreed case definition for NEC. Absence of an accepted, evidence-based case definition is problematic and a major challenge to advancing NEC research.[1-3]

The clinical presentation of NEC is often nonspecific, making the diagnosis of less severe disease even more uncertain. Even the widely accepted pathognomonic features of pneumatosis and portal venous gas occur late in disease and can be subject to interobserver variability.[4-6] Features such as "tenderness" can be difficult especially if infants are on intravenous sedation and pain relief; discoloration can be subjective. Even in the authors' population study conducted in England, in which they applied a more stringent definition, "severe NEC" defined as NEC confirmed at laparotomy, histology, or postmortem, or for whom cause of death was NEC, the authors acknowledge that opinions on whether to proceed to surgery, and whether an infant is too sick for surgery, can be variable.[7] Around two-thirds of very preterm infants receive at least one episode of medical management for presumed NEC, but whether they truly have the disease is uncertain.

A case definition that discriminates well between infants with and without NEC is needed for reliable surveillance, quality improvement, and clinical trials. Without a consistently applied case definition, it remains a challenge to synthesize results of clinical trials, progress preventive and therapeutic research, determine true disease burden, and perform international comparisons. In epidemiologic studies in high-income countries, the most commonly applied case definition is Bell's staging,[8-10] followed by the Vermont Oxford Network definition.[11] Other definitions include Bell's stage 1 to 3,[12] the definition from the Centers for Disease Control and Prevention,[13] and the International Classification for Diseases 10, although this is a code rather than a definition.[14] A combination of clinical and radiological signs specified by study authors is also used with some more stringent than others.[15-18] The wide range of definitions used for case ascertainment limits the extent to which the data can reliably be compared and pooled nationally and internationally. Bell's criteria, the most widely used, were devised by a surgeon in the 1970s as criteria to guide surgical management *after* the diagnosis was made. Although never intended for this purpose, it has since been modified and adopted as a case definition.[8,9] An additional source of variation is that many studies define NEC using Bell's staging but include different stages: Bell's stage 1 includes nonspecific findings such as feeding intolerance and abdominal distension; stage 2 requires radiographic findings of pneumatosis intestinalis and/or portal venous gas; stage 3 includes a perforated viscus, and infants with SIP managed with peritoneal drains without a laparotomy may be erroneously categorized under Bell's stage IIIb. Controversies exist on whether SIP is a separate entity to NEC, and how SIP is differentiated from NEC.[2] Therefore, "NEC" datasets may include infants with such other diagnoses. It is uncertain whether NEC now seen in extremely preterm infants, who previously did not survive, is the same disease used in the development of Bell's criteria. Furthermore, few definitions used are evidence based, are validated, or incorporate gestational age (GA) at birth, even though this is known to influence both risk and clinical presentation of NEC.[19] Sharma and colleagues[19] found that less mature infants were less likely to present with pneumatosis, bloody stool, and portal venous gas, and more likely to present with distension, ileus, and pneumoperitoneum compared with term infants with NEC. In a large, whole population surveillance study in England, the authors confirmed GA-based variability in clinical signs. They also used the data acquired to develop a GA-specific NEC risk score and case definition.[1,7]

The need for additional molecular markers to improve early diagnosis of NEC is well recognized, and there has been some advance in this area. Several circulatory molecules have shown considerable promise, including proinflammatory cytokines (tumor necrosis factorα, interleukin-6 [IL-6], and IL-8).[20] Other potential biomarkers include those reflecting enterocyte injury or intestinal barrier impairment, such as intestinal fatty acid–binding protein, liver fatty acid–binding protein, fecal calprotectin, trefoil factor 3, and claudin-3.[21,22] However, these candidate biomarkers require validation in prospective studies. Until such time, there is a need for consistent application of an evidence-based NEC case-definition.

PAUCITY OF PRECLINICAL RESEARCH

There is good recognition of NEC risk factors, namely immaturity, growth restriction, and formula feeding, but the extent to which these endogenous and exogenous factors are implicated causally in pathogenesis is unclear. Etiologic factors include chronic and acute hypoxemia, mucosal injury and immaturity, intestinal ischemia, exposure to opportunistic pathogens, and alteration of the intestinal microbiome. Intrauterine, perinatal, and postnatal insults trigger the inflammatory cascade, resulting in intestinal barrier compromise and gut-origin bloodstream infection.[23–25] Preclinical research has to date not translated into preventive clinical strategies.

REGULATORY CHALLENGES

A graphic example of a major challenge in NEC research is the story of clinical trials of probiotics for NEC prevention. In a recent review, the authors identified a total of 46 randomized controlled trials (RCTs) of probiotics for NEC prevention that enrolled a total of 12,185 infants (submitted). Nevertheless, despite this time, effort, and cost, no probiotic is as yet licensed for NEC prevention. The regulation of probiotic products is made complicated because they are widely classified as food supplements and not as medical products, an issue that is likely to be the case for other commercial products and is an issue that calls for a new approach to regulation that addresses the specific needs of the newborn baby.

DISEASE RARITY

Although NEC can be devastating in impact, it is a rare disease. A rare disease is defined by the European Union as one that affects less than 5 in 10,000 of the population. Based on an incidence in infants less than 29 weeks' gestation of around 10%, the prevalence estimate for NEC is around 1.6 per 10,000 people.

NEC is thought to affect 10% to 15% of very low-birth-weight infants.[14,26,27] However, most studies are not population based and describe incidence rates for single or groups of tertiary referral centers, casting doubt on the validity of the figures. In a systematic review of NEC incidence that included 12 studies from 14 high-income countries, the authors identified a median (range) rate in babies born less than 32 weeks' gestation of 3% (2%–7%), but this varied with the definition used.[10] The incidence is higher the greater the degree of immaturity. In less than 28 weeks' GA, infants' incidence rates have been reported ranging from 2% in Japan,[28] 4% in Switzerland,[29] to 7% to 9% in Australia, Canada, and Italy.[30–32] In infants born between 28 and 31 weeks' gestation, reported incidence varies from 0.2% in Japan to 2% to 3% in the other countries. In a 2-year complete population study in England, the authors found that 531 (0.4%) of 118,073 infants (all GA) admitted to neonatal units developed the severest form of NEC confirmed by laparotomy, histology, or autopsy, or for whom NEC was the primary cause of death. Of the 531, 87% (462 infants) were born less than 32 weeks' GA, giving an incidence rate of 3.2% in this GA group.

The low absolute numbers of NEC necessitates large RCTs to achieve adequate statistical power to detect clinically relevant differences. Most RCTs to date have been underpowered to examine the impact of interventions on NEC reliably. The emergence of large databases worldwide, curated from a range of administrative and/or point-of-care routine electronic patient records, offers promising opportunity to strengthen NEC surveillance[33] and provide accurate baseline incidence data, necessary to design adequately powered RCTs. The incidence of NEC also varies with geographic location; for example, the incidence of NEC in the ProPrems trial in Australia and New Zealand, which included 1099 infants born less than 32-weeks' GA, was 4.4% (3.0–6.4),[34] compared with 10% in the Probiotics in Preterms trial conducted in South-East England, which included 1315 infants less than 31-weeks' GA.[35]

COST OF CLINICAL TRIALS

Clinical trials are expensive and increasing in cost. In a recent evaluation of 726 interventional trials conducted by 7 top biopharma companies from 2010 to 2015, the median cost of conducting a study from protocol approval to final report was US$3.4 million for phase 1 trials, $8.6 million for phase 2 trials, and $21.4 million for phase 3 trials.[36] It is well recognized that the newborn market is limited, and industry contribution to clinical trials in the pediatric population is small, which led to the introduction of incentives in the United States and Europe to promote industry involvement in pediatric trials in the form of the Paediatric Regulation in the European Union,[37] which came into force in 2007 and the US Best Pharmaceuticals for Children Act in 2002 and the Pediatric Research Equity Act in 2003 (both amended in 2007).[38] The success of these incentivization schemes has been tangible but limited; hence, the authors suggest that future approaches to reduce the cost of neonatal trials might usefully address ways of strengthening international collaborations across public, charity, and industry sector funders.

QUALITY OF CLINICAL TRIALS

Many clinical trials have major methodological shortcomings; for example, in the example of probiotic research referred to above, the quality of trials was highly variable. Many studies were unregistered, and there was uncertainty regarding blinding, concealment of treatment allocation, type of randomization, and postrandomization exclusions. Despite acknowledged relevance and importance, few neonatal trials incorporate adequate long-term follow-up to gauge the impact of interventions on later functional outcomes. Too many neonatal trials rely on proxy or surrogate outcomes of uncertain relevance to later functional health measures. There is also considerable variation in the types of outcomes that investigators assess and report which poses a serious hindrance to pooling data in systematic reviews and meta-analyses. Initiatives to harmonize approaches and develop core outcome sets are important markers of early progress in this area.[39,40] Other work underway aims to improve standards in pediatric research.[41]

CLINICIAN BIAS

Clinicians frequently have strong preferences for particular approaches to neonatal care, and there is evidence that they retain these even when presented with a summary of existing evidence that indicates no clear benefit from any approach, which has potential to be a major barrier to delivering clinical trials. However, reassuringly, in a recent survey of UK clinicians, two-thirds of respondents expressed willingness to recruit babies to a proposed trial, despite expressing strong personal preferences.[42]

THE WAY FORWARD

In summary, there are several factors that make progressing NEC research difficult. The disease is variable in presentation. There are difficulties in making a precise diagnosis, and a reliable agreed case definition is currently lacking. There is a paucity of preclinical research to identify etiologic targets. The rarity of severe disease mandates collaboration across national and international boundaries to deliver studies with adequate power to address important outcomes. There may be reluctance of clinicians to randomize patients. The cost of clinical trials, including long-term outcome ascertainment, is a major challenge. There are insufficiently defined requirements for the licensing of nonpharmaceutical products, and need for closer parent-public involvement.

The authors suggest that international collaboration to address the challenges in NEC research offers the best way forward. They propose this might involve establishing a consortium of academic and clinical units, to address specific areas of need. Preclinical research is required to identify etiologic and effector pathways. Collaboration would facilitate, for example, the establishment of an international cohort study to identify and test candidate biomarkers of disease risk, diagnosis, and prognosis. Clinicians could assist by undertaking to record individual clinical signs, radiological, and laboratory parameters that could then contribute to sophisticated analyses using a variety of case definitions and test their predictive value against a gold standard, an approach the authors used in a recent whole population study.[7]

For treatment and clinical management approaches that are established components of accepted practice, but where the evidence based is lacking or insufficient, there is a strong case to be made for offering randomization using an opt-out process, as an accepted approach and standard of care.[43,44] Examples of uncertainties pertinent to NEC include the role of bovine-origin fortifier in increasing risk, the protective effect of hydrolyzed formulas, and the optimum feed after surgery. The incorporation of randomization and data collection into routine care offers enormous opportunity to realize the potential of deriving "real-world evidence" from "real-world data."

Finally, there is clear need to engage with regulators, industry, parents, and the public to foster collaboration and widen perspectives when addressing these many challenges. C-Path has established such a collaboration, the International Neonatal Consortium, for the specific purpose of establishing a defined regulatory path for evaluating the safety and effectiveness of therapies for neonates.[45]

Best practices

What is current best practice for necrotizing enterocolitis?

Current best practice for prevention and treatment are (i) being aware of infants at high risk; (ii) having a high degree of vigilance; (iii) meticulous supportive management; (iv) close collaboration between medical and surgical teams; and (v) supporting high-quality national and international research endeavor.

What changes in current practice are likely to change outcomes?

Many preventive and therapeutic options have been investigated or remain under investigation, but there is little high-quality evidence to guide management. A major area of potential benefit is to investigate whether an exclusive human milk diet, or avoidance of cow-milk products, protects against the disease. There have been several small trials with inconclusive results, but no adequately powered clinical trials addressing these research questions.

Summary statement

Because cause and pathophysiology, and preventive and therapeutic regimens, remain largely unknown, and severe necrotizing enterocolitis is a rare disease, close collaboration between researchers (clinical and preclinical), clinicians, funders, regulators, and parents, to deliver high-quality, adequately powered clinical trials nationally and internationally, and develop and test potential therapies, represents the approach most likely to reduce the burden of this devastating disease.

REFERENCES

1. Battersby C, Longford N, Costeloe K, et al, for the UK Neonatal Collaborative Necrotising Enterocolitis Study Group. Development of a gestational age-specific case definition for neonatal necrotizing enterocolitis. JAMA Pediatr 2017;171: 256–63.

2. Gordon PV, Swanson JR, Attridge JT, et al. Emerging trends in acquired neonatal intestinal disease: is it time to abandon Bell's criteria? J Perinatol 2007;27:661–71.

3. Gordon PV, Swanson JR, MacQueen BC, et al. A critical question for NEC researchers: can we create a consensus definition of NEC that facilitates research progress? Semin Perinatol 2017;41:7–14.

4. Tam AL, Camberos A, Applebaum H. Surgical decision making in necrotizing enterocolitis and focal intestinal perforation: predictive value of radiologic findings. J Pediatr Surg 2002;37:1688–91.

5. Rehan VK, Seshia MM, Johnston B, et al. Observer variability in interpretation of abdominal radiographs of infants with suspected necrotizing enterocolitis. Clin Pediatr (Phila) 1999;38:637–43.

6. Mata AG, Rosengart RM. Interobserver variability in the radiographic diagnosis of necrotizing enterocolitis. Pediatrics 1980;66:68–71.
7. Battersby C, Longford N, Mandalia S, et al, UK Neonatal Collaborative Necrotising Enterocolitis (UKNC-NEC) Study Group. Incidence and enteral feed antecedents of severe neonatal necrotising enterocolitis across neonatal networks in England, 2012-13: a whole-population surveillance study. Lancet Gastroenterol Hepatol 2017;2:43–51.
8. Kliegman RM, Walsh MC. Neonatal necrotizing enterocolitis: pathogenesis, classification, and spectrum of illness. Curr Probl Pediatr 1987;17:213–88.
9. Bell MJ, Ternberg JL, Feigin RD, et al. Neonatal necrotizing enterocolitis. Therapeutic decisions based upon clinical staging. Ann Surg 1978;187:1–7.
10. Battersby C, Santhalingam T, Costeloe K, et al. Incidence of neonatal necrotising enterocolitis in high-income countries: a systematic review. Arch Dis Child Fetal Neonatal Ed 2018;103:F182–9.
11. Vermont Oxford Network (VON). In: Vermont oxford network database manual of operations: part 2: data definitions and data forms for infants born in 2013. 17th edition (R Release). Burlington, VT: Vermont Oxford Network; 2012.
12. Tommiska V, Heinonen K, Ikonen S, et al. A National short-term follow-up study of extremely low birth weight infants born in finland in 1996–1997. Pediatrics 2001; 107:e2.
13. Leistner R, Piening B, Gastmeier P, et al. Nosocomial infections in very low birthweight infants in Germany: current data from the National Surveillance System NEO-KISS. Klin Padiatr 2013;225:75–80.
14. Ahle M, Drott P, Andersson RE. Epidemiology and trends of necrotizing enterocolitis in Sweden: 1987-2009. Pediatrics 2013;132:e443–51.
15. Kastenberg ZJ, Lee HC, Profit J, et al. Effect of deregionalized care on mortality in very low-birth-weight infants with necrotizing enterocolitis. JAMA Pediatr 2015; 169:26–32.
16. Fitzgibbons SC, Ching Y, Yu D, et al. Mortality of necrotizing enterocolitis expressed by birth weight categories. J Pediatr Surg 2009;44:1072–5.
17. Youn YA, Kim E-K, Kim SY. Necrotizing enterocolitis among very-low-birth-weight infants in Korea. J Korean Med Sci 2015;30(Suppl 1):S75–80.
18. Wojkowska-Mach J, Rozanska A, Borszewska-Kornacka M, et al. Necrotising enterocolitis in preterm infants: epidemiology and antibiotic consumption in the Polish neonatology network neonatal intensive care units in 2009. PLoS One 2014;9:e92865.
19. Sharma R, Hudak ML, Tepas JJ III, et al. Impact of gestational age on the clinical presentation and surgical outcome of necrotizing enterocolitis. J Perinatol 2006; 26:342–7.
20. Niemarkt HJ, de Meij TG, van de Velde ME, et al. Necrotizing enterocolitis: a clinical review on diagnostic biomarkers and the role of the intestinal microbiota. Inflamm Bowel Dis 2015;21:436–44.
21. Ng PC. Biomarkers of necrotising enterocolitis. Semin Fetal Neonatal Med 2014; 19:33–8.
22. Thuijls G, Derikx JPM, van Wijck K, et al. Non-invasive markers for early diagnosis and determination of the severity of necrotizing enterocolitis. Ann Surg 2010;251: 1174–80.
23. Neu J. Necrotizing enterocolitis: the mystery goes on. Neonatology 2014;106: 289–95.
24. Neu J, Pammi M. Pathogenesis of NEC: impact of an altered intestinal microbiome. Semin Perinatol 2017;41:29–35.

25. Denning TL, Bhatia AM, Kane AF, et al. Pathogenesis of NEC: role of the innate and adaptive immune response. Semin Perinatol 2017;41:15–28.

26. Stoll BJ, Hansen NI, Bell EF, et al. Trends in care practices, morbidity, and mortality of extremely preterm neonates, 1993-2012. JAMA 2015;314:1039–51.

27. Yee WH, Soraisham AS, Shah VS, et al. Incidence and timing of presentation of necrotizing enterocolitis in preterm infants. Pediatrics 2012;129:e298–304.

28. Isayama T, Lee SK, Mori R, et al. Comparison of mortality and morbidity of very low birth weight infants between Canada and Japan. Pediatrics 2012;130: e957–65.

29. Chen F, Bajwa NM, Rimensberger PC, et al, Swiss Neonatal Network. Thirteen-year mortality and morbidity in preterm infants in Switzerland. Arch Dis Child Fetal Neonatal Ed 2016;101:F377–83.

30. Hossain S, Shah PS, Ye XY, et al. Outcome comparison of very preterm infants cared for in the neonatal intensive care units in Australia and New Zealand and in Canada. J Paediatr Child Health 2015;51:881–8.

31. Isayama T, Shah PS, Ye XY, et al. Adverse impact of maternal cigarette smoking on preterm infants: a population-based cohort study. Am J Perinatol 2015;32: 1105–11.

32. Gagliardi L, Bellu R, Cardilli V, et al. Necrotising enterocolitis in very low birth weight infants in Italy: incidence and non-nutritional risk factors. J Pediatr Gastroenterol Nutr 2008;47:206–10.

33. Statnikov Y, Ibrahim B, Modi N. A systematic review of administrative and clinical databases of infants admitted to neonatal units. Arch Dis Child Fetal Neonatal Ed 2017;102:F270–6.

34. Jacobs SE, Tobin JM, Opie GF, et al, ProPrems Study Group. Probiotic effects on late-onset sepsis in very preterm infants: a randomized controlled trial. Pediatrics 2013;132:1055–62.

35. Costeloe K, Hardy P, Juszczak E, et al, Probiotics in Preterm Infants Study Collaborative Group. Bifidobacterium breve BBG-001 in very preterm infants: a randomised controlled phase 3 trial. Lancet 2016;387:649–60.

36. Martin L, Hutchens M, Hawkins C, et al. How much do clinical trials cost? Nat Rev Drug Discov 2017;16:381–2.

37. European medicines Agency 2007 The European paediatric initiative: History of the Paediatric Regulation. Available at: http://www.ema.europa.eu/docs/en_GB/document_library/Other/2009/09/WC500003693.pdf. Accessed April 6, 2018.

38. Department of Health and Human Services Food and Drug Administration 2016 Best Pharmaceuticals for Children Act and Pediatric Research Equity Act Status Report to Congress. Available at: https://www.fda.gov/downloads/science research/specialtopics/pediatrictherapeuticsresearch/ucm509815.pdf. Accessed April 6, 2018.

39. Webbe J, Brunton G, Ali S, et al. Implementing and disseminating a core outcome set for neonatal medicine. BMJ Paediatr Open 2017;1:e000048.

40. Duffy J, Rolph R, Gale C, et al, International Collaboration to Harmonise Outcomes in Pre-eclampsia (iHOPE). Core outcome sets in women's and newborn health: a systematic review. BJOG 2017;124:1481–9.

41. Offringa M, Needham AC, Chan WW, StaR Child Health Group. StaR Child Health: improving global standards for child health research. Early Hum Dev 2013;89:861–4.

42. Mills L, Modi N. Clinician enteral feeding preferences for very preterm babies in the UK. Arch Dis Child Fetal Neonatal Ed 2015;100:F372–3.

43. Gale C, Hyde MJ, Modi N. WHEAT trial development group Research ethics com-mittee decision-making in relation to an efficient neonatal trial. Arch Dis Child Fetal Neonatal Ed 2017;102:F291–8.
44. Gale C, Modi N. WHEAT trial development group Neonatal randomised point-of-care trials are feasible and acceptable in the UK: results from two national sur-veys. Arch Dis Child Fetal Neonatal Ed 2016;101:F86–7.
45. International Neonatal Consortium. Available at: https://c-path.org/programs/inc/. Accessed April 6, 2018.

Necrotizing Enterocolitis Pathophysiology

How Microbiome Data Alter Our Understanding

Christina S. Kim, MD*, Erika C. Claud, MD

KEYWORDS

• Necrotizing enterocolitis • Microbiome • Antibiotic stewardship • Genomics

KEY POINTS

- Alterations in the balance of the commensal gut microbiome in neonates may be related to risk for necrotizing enterocolitis.
- The newborn gut microbiome seems to develop in the setting of both prenatal and postnatal exposures.
- Colonization of the gut microbiome occurs in a relatively orderly and stepwise process.
- The preterm intestinal microbiota seems to differ from term infants and points to the relevance of the microbiome in the development of necrotizing enterocolitis.

INTRODUCTION

The pathophysiology of necrotizing enterocolitis (NEC) is a complex and multifactorial process that has been the topic of many areas of research in neonatology. NEC is a significant cause of morbidity and mortality in premature neonates,[1,2] as well as a major player in the economics of hospital care and medicine.[3,4] In North America, NEC affects approximately 7% of very low birth weight infants (birth weight of ≤1500 g), with as many as 20% to 30% of these patients dying of this major gastrointestinal disease.[5,6] Survivors of NEC are at risk for a range of complications, including short gut syndrome and neurodevelopmental delays.[7] Although the exact mechanism of NEC remains unknown, many aspects of the disease have been observed and discussed in literature, including the role of the gut microbiome as it relates to the evolution of NEC. Research in this area is expanding and, with advances in bacterial analysis, our understanding of the relationship between the microbiome and NEC continues to grow.

Disclosure Statement: The authors have no financial interests to disclose.
Neonatology, Department of Pediatrics, University of Chicago, 5841 South Maryland Avenue, MC 6060, Chicago, IL 60637, USA
* Corresponding author.
E-mail address: christina.kim2@uchospitals.edu

Clin Perinatol 46 (2019) 29–38
https://doi.org/10.1016/j.clp.2018.10.003
0095-5108/19/© 2018 Elsevier Inc. All rights reserved.

NEONATAL MICROBIOME

The human microbiome is considered the "sum of microbial life living in and on the human body."[8] Its study has been largely facilitated by advances in the field of genomics, and research continues to show the importance between the microbiome and its host. The microbiome seems to play a role in a broad range of essential functions, including metabolism, nutrition, and the immune system. It begins to develop from birth, and as discussed elsewhere in this article, perhaps even earlier in utero, and continues to evolve throughout life to maintain homeostasis with its host.[9] The gut microbiome is of particular interest in neonatal research because there seem to be multiple identifiable and modifiable factors that may alter both the establishment and development of this commensal community of bacteria.

TECHNIQUES IN MICROBIOME ANALYSIS

Recent advances in research surrounding microbiome analyses have been spurred on by the increasing use of non–culture-based techniques in the evaluation of intestinal bacteria. Because many bacteria found in stool samples cannot be analyzed using traditional culture-based methods, the role of genomic sequencing has opened up this area of research. Two of the more commonly used approaches are 16S rRNA sequencing and metagenomics. The 16s rRNA component of ribosomal RNA is of particular usefulness for studies related to the microbiome, because genes encoding this region can be highly conserved or variable and therefore facilitate taxonomic classification of bacteria.[10] Metagenomic sequencing may provide even more information as to function, because this approach is not limited to the 16s rRNA regions. These methods allow for a more comprehensive approach to the analysis of intestinal microbial communities.

ROLE AND DEVELOPMENT OF THE COMMENSAL MICROBIOME

The human gastrointestinal tract assumes many critical roles, including providing a connection between the internal and external environments of the body. This large immune organ must find the delicate balance between protecting against harmful pathogens, while serving as host to commensal bacteria.[11] This paradigm seems especially relevant to the pathogenesis of NEC, in that there seems to be an association between the perturbation of the makeup and homeostasis of the gut microbiome and the uncontrolled inflammation seen in NEC. Commensal bacteria are important in a number of gastrointestinal functions, including digestion[12] and the adaptive immune response.[13] Therefore, the establishment of the host microbiome in a newborn is a delicate and essential process in their development.

Intrauterine Origin of the Microbiome

Although there remains debate regarding exactly when the newborn gut begins to acquire commensal bacteria, there is increasing evidence that this process may begin in utero. In a study by Ardissone and colleagues,[14] meconium was collected from infants 23 to 41 weeks of gestation, analyzed using 16s rRNA sequencing methods, and compared with previously studied bacterial profiles of amniotic fluid. The investigators found multiple bacterial genera in common between the meconium and amniotic fluid. This idea that the maternal uterine environment may affect the infant gut microbiome is of particular interest when looking at studies that demonstrate microbial dysbiosis in mothers with preterm premature rupture of membranes (PPROM). In a study by Baldwin and colleagues,[15] investigators attempted to characterize amniotic fluid discharge and the vaginal microbiome by taking serial vaginal swabs from the onset of PPROM until delivery. The samples were analyzed using 16s rRNA sequencing, and results showed that, although there was substantial variation between the microbiomes of PPROM subjects, overall trends indicated that the bacterial makeup of the vagina and amniotic fluid discharge was significantly influenced by exposure to latency antibiotics. This study showed the persistent microbial dysbiosis present in mothers with PPROM from onset until delivery and, if indeed there is a connection between amniotic fluid and the infant microbiome, then antenatal antibiotic exposure may play a role in the development of the neonatal gut microbiota.

Other studies have also identified microbial DNA sequences in meconium samples of newborns, supporting the idea of an intrauterine origin of the gut microbiome.[16,17] Further corroboration of this idea is provided by research looking at the presence and profile of bacteria in placental cultures,[18] although these studies do not specifically look at any potential relationship between the microbial makeup of the placenta compared with the newborn gastrointestinal tract. In contrast, a study by Lauder and colleagues[19] concluded that a distinctive microbial profile could not be found in placental samples when compared with contamination controls, countering the idea of a placental microbiome. Ultimately, these studies show that the role the intrauterine environment plays in the development of the neonatal microbiome seems to be relevant and requires further study and analysis.

Extrauterine Development of the Microbiome

Many factors seem to play a role in the development of the newborn gut microbiome in the extrauterine environment, including the mode of delivery (cesarean vs vaginal) and the type of enteral feeds (formula vs breast milk).[20,21] Preterm infants admitted to a neonatal intensive care unit encounter an additional set of variables in that they may be exposed to certain medications (namely antibiotics), require feeding tubes, and have enteral feeds introduced more slowly. The intensive care environment itself may also influence a patient's microbiome, from hand hygiene practices to central line care.[22]

Mode of delivery

The cesarean delivery rate in the United States in 2016 was 31.9%.[23] Although this is the lowest rate since 2007, cesarean deliveries remain a significant portion of overall births, and several studies have shown differences in the microbiome of newborns after cesarean and vaginal deliveries.[24] In a more recent non–culture-based study by Dominguez-Bello and colleagues,[25] investigators showed that samples taken from the skin, oral mucosa, and nasopharyngeal aspirates of newborns delivered vaginally reflected their mother's vaginal microbiota, namely *Lactobacillus*, *Prevotella*, or *Sneathia* species. In contrast, samples taken from newborns delivered via cesarean section showed bacteria more commonly found on the skin surface, including *Staphylococcus*, *Corynebacterium*, and *Propionibacterium* species. Although bacteria related to cesarean deliveries seems to have more pathogenic potential to the host, there have been no studies showing an association between delivery mode and the development of NEC to date.

Enteral exposures, including type of feeds and probiotics

Multiple studies have shown that an exclusive human milk diet decreases the incidence of both medical and surgical NEC in preterm infants.[26–29] The understanding of the benefits of human milk are also reflected in the American Academy of Pediatrics Policy Statement from 2017, which recommends donor milk for preterm infants (particularly those ≤1500 g) when the mother's milk is not available.[30] Many components of human milk seem to be related to the decreased incidence of NEC, including immunoglobulins, lactoferrin, lysozyme, and human milk oligosaccharides. Human milk oligosaccharides make up the third largest component of human milk and may play a significant role in the development of the newborn microbiome[31] through selective consumption by commensal gut bacteria.[32] In healthy term infants who are receiving an exclusive human milk diet, *Bifidobacteria* and *Bacteroidetes* are able to thrive secondary to their ability to digest human milk oligosaccharides, whereas pathogenic bacteria such as *Enterobacteriaceae* are unable to use human milk oligosaccharides to promote their proliferation.[33] Interestingly, the administration of probiotics containing *Bifidobacteria* to preterm infants leads to a decreased risk of NEC.[34]

The idea that the gut microbiome may be altered by certain enteral exposures is also reflected in research surrounding probiotics. Probiotics may be a way in which beneficial commensal strains of certain bacteria can be introduced into an infant's gut microbiome to potentially provide protection against inflammation and ultimately NEC.[11] A metaanalysis of 20 randomized, controlled trials demonstrated that probiotics decrease both severe NEC and all-cause mortality.[35] Although the 2 most commonly used probiotic agents are *Bifidobacteria* and *Lactobacillus*, the optimal type of probiotic supplement has not yet been determined,[36] and concerns for the risk of infection and sepsis continue. The complicated nature of the use of probiotics as a therapeutic agent is also reflected in the intricate balance of the gut microbiome. Maintaining the complex homeostasis of the infant intestinal microbiota may not be as simple as exposing the gastrointestinal tract to 1 or 2 genera of beneficial bacteria, and may require a more wholistic approach to the microbiome.

Antibiotics and other medications

It is often standard practice in the neonatal intensive care unit to initiate empiric antibiotic therapy for preterm infants upon delivery for the potential for early-onset sepsis. Although the morbidity and mortality related to early-onset sepsis is high, the actual rate of early-onset sepsis is low at 0.98 per 1000 live births.[37] This finding supports the idea that the judicial use of antibiotics in certain lower risk preterm patients may be done safely, potentially allowing for the maintenance of the commensal gut microbiome in these infants. Multiple studies have shown an association between prolonged antibiotic therapy and an increased risk of NEC.[38–40] In a retrospective cohort analysis of extremely low birth weight infants, Cotten and colleagues[38] showed that prolonged empiric antibiotic therapy (started in the first 3 postnatal days with sterile culture results, ≥5 days' duration) was associated with an increased odds of NEC. Similarly, in a retrospective case-controlled study, Alexander and colleagues[40] showed that the duration of antibiotic therapy was associated with an increased risk of NEC in neonates without previous sepsis. Because it is generally understood that antibiotics cause alterations in the makeup of both commensal and pathogenic microbiota, these studies support the idea that variables (such as antibiotic exposure) that affect gut bacteria may also affect the pathogenesis of NEC.

Although there have not been many large cohort studies looking at the association between specific antibiotic regimens and their effects on the makeup of the gut microbiome, some smaller studies have shown interesting taxonomic patterns of the bacteria from neonatal stool samples in patients exposed to antibiotics.[41–43] In a study by Greenwood and colleagues,[41] investigators used 16s rRNA sequencing to show that early empiric antibiotic use in preterm infants led to an increased abundance of *Enterobacter*, lower bacterial diversity of the gut microbiome overall in the second and third weeks of life, and more cases of NEC. The initial decrease in bacterial diversity after empiric antibiotic exposure (in this case, ampicillin and gentamicin) in this study contrasts with a study done by Tanaka and colleagues,[42] which showed no significant differences of the gut microbiota in infants born at 36 weeks of gestation or later in the first month after therapy with oral cephalexin. Although the 2 studies are difficult to compare owing to multiple differing variables, they both illustrate the fact that larger studies are required to look at factors such as specific antibiotic classes and route of administration in relation to the gut microbiome, and ultimately the risk of NEC.[44] Similar to antibiotics, H2-blocker medications such as ranitidine have been associated with an increased risk of NEC.[45,46] As in the study from Greenwood and colleagues,[41] Gupta and colleagues[47] also used 16s rRNA sequencing to show lower microbial diversity and increase in relative abundance of *Enterobacteriaceae* in stool samples taken from preterm infants exposed to H2-blockers.

INTESTINAL MICROBIOTA AND INFLAMMATION

The intestinal mucosa carries out multiple complex functions, including serving as a first line barrier defense from potential pathogens, as well as modulation of the innate immune system.[13,48,49] Both commensal and pathogenic gut bacteria contain microbial-associated molecular patterns (MAMPs)[50] that are recognized by specific pattern recognition receptors present on the intestinal mucosa. Microbial cell wall products such as lipopolysaccharides and peptidoglycans may serve as MAMPs that are recognized by pattern recognition receptors on human intestinal cells, such as Toll-like receptors (TLRs). These intricate interactions lead to signaling pathways involved in critical gastrointestinal tract functions such as homeostasis and inflammatory effects.[11] The makeup of the gut microbiome is therefore extremely relevant as certain MAMPs present on specific bacteria may activate versus deactivate inflammatory pathways, which in turn may affect the risk of NEC.

The relationship between MAMPs and their TLRs is highly specific.[51] A well-known signaling pathway that may be involved in the pathogenesis of NEC is the activation of TLR-4 by lipopolysaccharides present on gram-negative bacteria.[52,53] Studies have shown that TLR-4 is involved in the phagocytosis and translocation of these gram-negative bacteria across the intestinal mucosal barrier.[54] The activation of receptors like TLR-4 can also lead to the activation of nuclear factor κB and caspases, which can then lead to the induction of proinflammatory cytokines such as certain tumor necrosis factors and interleukins.[11] It has been postulated that an end result of this pathway may lead to the development of NEC.[55] Although this pathway is just an example of a component of the likely pathophysiology of NEC, it illustrates the overarching idea that patterns of microbial colonization in the preterm gut are related to the expression of regulation of such pathways, and are therefore correlated to the risk of NEC.

GUT BACTERIAL ASSEMBLY IN PRETERM INFANTS

As mentioned, there seem to be many factors that play into the development of the newborn gut microbiome. There have been a number of studies looking at the intestinal microbiota of preterm infants without NEC using either 16s rRNA or metagenomic sequencing.[56–61] Overall, the data from these studies support the paradigm that colonization of the newborn gut occurs in a relatively orderly process. In a study by La Rosa and colleagues,[61] investigators showed a reproducible pattern in the evolution of the preterm gut microbiome in infants without NEC. Initial samples were predominantly of the Bacilli class (gram-positive cocci such as *Staphylococci*, *Streptococci*, and *Enterococci*). These were then overtaken by gram-negative facultative bacteria of the Gammaproteobacteria class, and this second surge was then counterbalanced by about 20 days of life with *Clostridia*. An additional interesting observation by the investigators of this study was that the overall bacterial composition of preterm infant (median gestational age of 27 weeks) stool samples studied differed from the intestinal bacterial composition that would be expected in term infants, older children, and adults. The preterm stool samples had higher percentages of Gammaproteobacteria and fewer obligate anaerobes. Although direct causality between factors such as a specific class of bacteria or timing of postnatal predominance of a certain group of bacteria and NEC has not been shown, it is interesting to note that the preterm infant gut microbiome differs in composition with term newborns.

ANALYSIS OF INTESTINAL MICROBIOME IN INFANTS WITH NECROTIZING ENTEROCOLITIS

A number of studies comparing the intestinal microbiota of preterm infants with and without NEC have pointed toward an association between Gammaproteobacteria and an increased risk for NEC.[56,60,62] These data correlate with what has been mentioned previously regarding TLRs and the activation of proinflammatory pathways by MAMPs presents on gram-negative bacteria. Although these data are compelling, research shows that the pathogenesis of NEC is extremely complex, and studies using non–culture-based bacterial sequencing techniques continue to produce highly variable results. Some investigators postulate that the wide variation in microbiota composition seen across different studies may be center specific.[63] Other investigators point to limitations in the sample size of most studies, and the difficulties inherit in capturing data related to such a dynamic disease process. This finding is reflected in those studies showing the progression of intestinal bacterial colonization of the preterm gut, and the seemingly abrupt shifts that can occur from phase to phase.[61]

SUMMARY

NEC is a devastating disease that continues to play a significant role in the mortality and morbidity of preterm infants. Although many layers of the pathophysiology of this complex gastrointestinal disorder have been studied, the role of the intestinal microbiome and the evolution of NEC seems to be one of the most promising areas of research. Newer genetic sequencing techniques have allowed for a more elegant, specific, and practical approach to the study of microbiota, and these findings must continue to be discussed and applied to what is already known about the disease. The idea of the intestinal microbiome playing a role in the development of NEC appears to be significant starting even in utero, and may be related to many of the postnatal variables that have been shown to relate to NEC, including type of enteral feeds and antibiotic exposure. There continues to be a high degree of variability in the genetic sequencing studies of the intestinal microbiota, stressing the importance of continued research in this field.

REFERENCES

1. Neu J, Walker WA. Necrotizing enterocolitis. N Engl J Med 2011;364(3):255–64.
2. Lin PW, Stoll BJ. Necrotising enterocolitis. Lancet 2006;368(9543):1271–83.
3. Stey A, Barnert ES, Tseng CH, et al. Outcomes and costs of surgical treatments of necrotizing enterocolitis. Pediatrics 2015;135(5):e1190–7.

4. Bisquera JA, Cooper TR, Berseth CL. Impact of necrotizing enterocolitis on length of stay and hospital charges in very low birth weight infants. Pediatrics 2002;109(3):423–8.

5. Fitzgibbons SC, Ching Y, Yu D, et al. Mortality of necrotizing enterocolitis expressed by birth weight categories. J Pediatr Surg 2009;44(6):1072–5 [discussion: 1075–6].

6. Holman RC, Stoll BJ, Curns AT, et al. Necrotising enterocolitis hospitalisations among neonates in the United States. Paediatr Perinat Epidemiol 2006;20(6): 498–506.

7. Hintz SR, Kendrick DE, Stoll BJ, et al. Neurodevelopmental and growth outcomes of extremely low birth weight infants after necrotizing enterocolitis. Pediatrics 2005;115(3):696–703.

8. Fricke WF. The more the merrier? Reduced fecal microbiota diversity in preterm infants treated with antibiotics. J Pediatr 2014;165(1):8–10.

9. Gritz EC, Bhandari V. The human neonatal gut microbiome: a brief review. Front Pediatr 2015;3:17.

10. Torrazza RM, Neu J. The altered gut microbiome and necrotizing enterocolitis. Clin Perinatol 2013;40(1):93–108.

11. Patel RM, Denning PW. Intestinal microbiota and its relationship with necrotizing enterocolitis. Pediatr Res 2015;78(3):232–8.

12. Guarner F, Malagelada JR. Gut flora in health and disease. Lancet 2003; 361(9356):512–9.

13. Round JL, Mazmanian SK. The gut microbiota shapes intestinal immune responses during health and disease. Nat Rev Immunol 2009;9(5):313–23.

14. Ardissone AN, de la Cruz DM, Davis-Richardson AG, et al. Meconium microbiome analysis identifies bacteria correlated with premature birth. PLoS One 2014;9(3):e90784.

15. Baldwin EA, Walther-Antonio M, MacLean AM, et al. Persistent microbial dysbiosis in preterm premature rupture of membranes from onset until delivery. PeerJ 2015;3:e1398.

16. Mshvildadze M, Neu J, Shuster J, et al. Intestinal microbial ecology in premature infants assessed with non-culture-based techniques. J Pediatr 2010;156(1):20–5.

17. Heida FH, van Zoonen A, Hulscher JBF, et al. A necrotizing enterocolitis-associated gut microbiota is present in the meconium: results of a prospective study. Clin Infect Dis 2016;62(7):863–70.

18. Aagaard K, Ma J, Antony KM, et al. The placenta harbors a unique microbiome. Sci Transl Med 2014;6(237):237ra65.

19. Lauder AP, Roche AM, Sherrill-Mix S, et al. Comparison of placenta samples with contamination controls does not provide evidence for a distinct placenta microbiota. Microbiome 2016;4(1):29.

20. Backhed F, Roswall J, Peng Y, et al. Dynamics and stabilization of the human gut microbiome during the first year of life. Cell Host Microbe 2015;17(5):690–703.

21. Palmer C, Bik EM, DiGiulio DB, et al. Development of the human infant intestinal microbiota. PLoS Biol 2007;5(7):e177.

22. Warner BB, Tarr PI. Necrotizing enterocolitis and preterm infant gut bacteria. Semin Fetal Neonatal Med 2016;21(6):394–9.

23. Martin JA, Hamilton BE, Osterman MJK, et al. Births: final data for 2016. Natl Vital Stat Rep 2018;67(1):1–55.

24. Neu J, Rushing J. Cesarean versus vaginal delivery: long-term infant outcomes and the hygiene hypothesis. Clin Perinatol 2011;38(2):321–31.

25. Dominguez-Bello MG, Costello EK, Contreras M, et al. Delivery mode shapes the acquisition and structure of the initial microbiota across multiple body habitats in newborns. Proc Natl Acad Sci U S A 2010;107(26):11971–5.
26. Lucas A, Cole TJ. Breast milk and neonatal necrotising enterocolitis. Lancet 1990; 336(8730):1519–23.
27. Sullivan S, Schanler RJ, Kim JH, et al. An exclusively human milk-based diet is associated with a lower rate of necrotizing enterocolitis than a diet of human milk and bovine milk-based products. J Pediatr 2010;156(4):562–567 e561.
28. Cristofalo EA, Schanler RJ, Blanco CL, et al. Randomized trial of exclusive human milk versus preterm formula diets in extremely premature infants. J Pediatr 2013; 163(6):1592–5.e1.
29. Kantorowska A, Wei JC, Cohen RS, et al. Impact of donor milk availability on breast milk use and necrotizing enterocolitis rates. Pediatrics 2016;137(3): e20153123.
30. Committee on Nutrition, Section on Breastfeeding, Committee on Fetus and Newborn. Donor human milk for the high-risk infant: preparation, safety, and usage options in the United States. Pediatrics 2017;139(1) [pii:e20163440].
31. Underwood MA, Gaerlan S, De Leoz ML, et al. Human milk oligosaccharides in premature infants: absorption, excretion, and influence on the intestinal microbiota. Pediatr Res 2015;78(6):670–7.
32. Sela DA, Mills DA. Nursing our microbiota: molecular linkages between bifidobacteria and milk oligosaccharides. Trends Microbiol 2010;18(7):298–307.
33. Yu ZT, Chen C, Newburg DS. Utilization of major fucosylated and sialylated human milk oligosaccharides by isolated human gut microbes. Glycobiology 2013;23(11):1281–92.
34. Deshpande G, Rao S, Patole S, et al. Updated meta-analysis of probiotics for preventing necrotizing enterocolitis in preterm neonates. Pediatrics 2010;125(5): 921–30.
35. AlFaleh K, Anabrees J. Probiotics for prevention of necrotizing enterocolitis in preterm infants. Cochrane Database Syst Rev 2014;(4):CD005496.
36. Wang Q, Dong J, Zhu Y. Probiotic supplement reduces risk of necrotizing enterocolitis and mortality in preterm very low-birth-weight infants: an updated meta-analysis of 20 randomized, controlled trials. J Pediatr Surg 2012;47(1):241–8.
37. Stoll BJ, Hansen NI, Sanchez PJ, et al. Early onset neonatal sepsis: the burden of group B Streptococcal and E. coli disease continues. Pediatrics 2011;127(5): 817–26.
38. Cotten CM, Taylor S, Stoll B, et al. Prolonged duration of initial empirical antibiotic treatment is associated with increased rates of necrotizing enterocolitis and death for extremely low birth weight infants. Pediatrics 2009;123(1):58–66.
39. Kuppala VS, Meinzen-Derr J, Morrow AL, et al. Prolonged initial empirical antibiotic treatment is associated with adverse outcomes in premature infants. J Pediatr 2011;159(5):720–5.
40. Alexander VN, Northrup V, Bizzarro MJ. Antibiotic exposure in the newborn intensive care unit and the risk of necrotizing enterocolitis. J Pediatr 2011;159(3): 392–7.
41. Greenwood C, Morrow AL, Lagomarcino AJ, et al. Early empiric antibiotic use in preterm infants is associated with lower bacterial diversity and higher relative abundance of Enterobacter. J Pediatr 2014;165(1):23–9.
42. Tanaka S, Kobayashi T, Songjinda P, et al. Influence of antibiotic exposure in the early postnatal period on the development of intestinal microbiota. FEMS Immunol Med Microbiol 2009;56(1):80–7.

43. Tagare A, Kadam S, Vaidya U, et al. Routine antibiotic use in preterm neonates: a randomised controlled trial. J Hosp Infect 2010;74(4):332–6.
44. Gibson MK, Crofts TS, Dantas G. Antibiotics and the developing infant gut microbiota and resistome. Curr Opin Microbiol 2015;27:51–6.
45. Guillet R, Stoll BJ, Cotten CM, et al. Association of H2-blocker therapy and higher incidence of necrotizing enterocolitis in very low birth weight infants. Pediatrics 2006;117(2):e137–42.
46. Terrin G, Passariello A, De Curtis M, et al. Ranitidine is associated with infections, necrotizing enterocolitis, and fatal outcome in newborns. Pediatrics 2012;129(1): e40–5.
47. Gupta RW, Tran L, Norori J, et al. Histamine-2 receptor blockers alter the fecal microbiota in premature infants. J Pediatr Gastroenterol Nutr 2013;56(4):397–400.
48. Sharma R, Young C, Neu J. Molecular modulation of intestinal epithelial barrier: contribution of microbiota. J Biomed Biotechnol 2010;2010:305879.
49. Murgas Torrazza R, Neu J. The developing intestinal microbiome and its relationship to health and disease in the neonate. J Perinatol 2011;31(Suppl 1):S29–34.
50. Rakoff-Nahoum S, Paglino J, Eslami-Varzaneh F, et al. Recognition of commensal microflora by toll-like receptors is required for intestinal homeostasis. Cell 2004; 118(2):229–41.
51. Rhee SH. Basic and translational understandings of microbial recognition by toll-like receptors in the intestine. J Neurogastroenterol Motil 2011;17(1):28–34.
52. Lu P, Sodhi CP, Hackam DJ. Toll-like receptor regulation of intestinal development and inflammation in the pathogenesis of necrotizing enterocolitis. Pathophysiology 2014;21(1):81–93.
53. Yazji I, Sodhi CP, Lee EK, et al. Endothelial TLR4 activation impairs intestinal microcirculatory perfusion in necrotizing enterocolitis via eNOS-NO-nitrite signaling. Proc Natl Acad Sci U S A 2013;110(23):9451–6.
54. Neal MD, Leaphart C, Levy R, et al. Enterocyte TLR4 mediates phagocytosis and translocation of bacteria across the intestinal barrier. J Immunol 2006;176(5): 3070–9.
55. Leaphart CL, Cavallo J, Gribar SC, et al. A critical role for TLR4 in the pathogenesis of necrotizing enterocolitis by modulating intestinal injury and repair. J Immunol 2007;179(7):4808–20.
56. Zhou Y, Shan G, Sodergren E, et al. Longitudinal analysis of the premature infant intestinal microbiome prior to necrotizing enterocolitis: a case-control study. PLoS One 2015;10(3):e0118632.
57. Ward DV, Scholz M, Zolfo M, et al. Metagenomic sequencing with strain-level resolution implicates uropathogenic E. coli in necrotizing enterocolitis and mortality in preterm infants. Cell Rep 2016;14(12):2912–24.
58. Sim K, Shaw AG, Randell P, et al. Dysbiosis anticipating necrotizing enterocolitis in very premature infants. Clin Infect Dis 2015;60(3):389–97.
59. Gibson MK, Wang B, Ahmadi S, et al. Developmental dynamics of the preterm infant gut microbiota and antibiotic resistome. Nat Microbiol 2016;1:16024.
60. Warner BB, Deych E, Zhou Y, et al. Gut bacteria dysbiosis and necrotising enterocolitis in very low birthweight infants: a prospective case-control study. Lancet 2016;387(10031):1928–36.
61. La Rosa PS, Warner BB, Zhou Y, et al. Patterned progression of bacterial populations in the premature infant gut. Proc Natl Acad Sci U S A 2014;111(34): 12522–7.

62. Wang Y, Hoenig JD, Malin KJ, et al. 16S rRNA gene-based analysis of fecal microbiota from preterm infants with and without necrotizing enterocolitis. ISME J 2009;3(8):944–54.
63. Taft DH, Ambalavanan N, Schibler KR, et al. Center variation in intestinal microbiota prior to late-onset sepsis in preterm infants. PLoS One 2015;10(6): e0130604.

Closing the Gap Between Recommended and Actual Human Milk Use for Fragile Infants

What Will It Take to Overcome Disparities?

Sheila M. Gephart, PhD, RN[a],*,
Katherine M. Newnam, PhD, RN, CPNP, NNP-BC, IBCLE[b]

KEYWORDS

- Necrotizing enterocolitis • Disparities • Very low birth weight infant • Human milk
- Human milk expression • Donor milk • Breastfeeding

KEY POINTS

- Human milk is recommended best care for fragile infants yet, access to human milk varies by neonatal intensive care unit and by race.
- Disparities surrounding human milk access may partially explain differences in rates of necrotizing enterocolitis across neonatal intensive care units.
- Quality improvement efforts to boost human milk exposure also reduce necrotizing enterocolitis rates.
- Effective quality improvement prioritizes early education and advocacy; lactation support for mothers to initiate, track, and sustain pumping; and staff education.
- Insights from broad-scale, effective quality improvement interventions, use of mobile health, and checklists could support consistency and close gaps.

Disclosure Statement: Dr S.M. Gephart received research funding from the Robert Wood Johnson Foundation Nurse Faculty Scholars Program (72112), the Agency for Healthcare Research and Quality (K08HS022908), and an express outreach award from the University of California, Los Angeles, Louise M. Darling Biomedical Library, headquarters for the National Network of Libraries of Medicine, Pacific Southwest Region (NNLM PSR). The content is solely the responsibility of the authors and does not necessarily represent the official views of the Agency for Healthcare Research and Quality, Robert Wood Johnson Foundation, or NNLM.

[a] Community and Health Systems Science Division, College of Nursing, The University of Arizona, PO Box 210203, Tucson, AZ 85721, USA; [b] College of Nursing, The University of Tennessee Knoxville, 1200 Volunteer Boulevard #361, Knoxville, TN 37996, USA
* Corresponding author.
E-mail address: gepharts@email.arizona.edu

Clin Perinatol 46 (2019) 39–50
https://doi.org/10.1016/j.clp.2018.09.003
0095-5108/19/© 2018 Elsevier Inc. All rights reserved.

As premature birth occurs at a rate of 1 in 8 US births, the challenge of reducing long-term morbidity for survivors persists. Among those born very low birth weight (ie, <1500 g), nearly one-third will experience serious complications.[1] Along with the impact on long-term health, neonatal complications dramatically increase the costs of care to the order of 4 to 7 times compared with infants who progress without them.[2] Yet, occurrence of complications varies widely from one neonatal intensive care unit (NICU) to another.[3–5] A chief threat to neonatal health is the challenge of necrotizing enterocolitis (NEC),[1] which is commonly described as multifactorial, acquired, inflammation driven, and characterized by dysbiosis and intestinal immaturity. This serious and potentially fatal intestinal disease involves widespread inflammatory activation, intestinal injury, and leads to systemic sepsis, particularly when the bowel wall is significantly compromised or ruptured in the most severe cases. NEC is among the primary reasons for neonatal emergency surgery and death among very low birth weight infants, but evidence suggests some risk factors may be partially modified. Leveraging consistent feeding guidelines and preferential use of human milk are critical to modify risk for NEC. This narrative review discusses human milk as medicine, its antiinflammatory components and composition, cost effectiveness, racial and NICU-level disparities influencing access, how to engage mothers, key lactation supports to promote use, and the effect of quality improvement interventions to boost human milk exposure.

HUMAN MILK AS MEDICINE

Human milk provides benefits to fragile infants that exceed the need for nutrition. Exclusive components within human milk promote the development of the immature immune system while reducing chronic inflammation, the primary challenge in fragile newborns. Many have begun describing human milk for the preterm infant as medicine and describe colostrum (the first milk produced by biological mothers; heretofore "mothers") as "liquid gold."[6] Most complications of prematurity have a component of inflammation in their causal pathways, including chronic lung disease, retinopathy of prematurity, white matter injury of the brain, and NEC.[7,8] Inflammation, a critical part of the infant's immune system, is the rapid activation of biochemical and cellular mechanisms in response to invasive organisms or tissue damage. This protective process is quickly activated through proinflammatory cytokines in the preterm infant, but is not well downregulated contributing to oxidative stress[9] and secondary tissue loss, negatively affecting these vulnerable systems.[10] Bioactive compounds in both maternal colostrum and mature human milk provide the infant with multiple cytokines, chemokines, growth factors, and immunoglobulins.[11] These factors support both anti-infectious and antiinflammatory properties, which aids in the regulation of the neonatal inflammatory response, reducing primary and secondary tissue loss.[12]

COST EFFECTIVENESS OF FEEDING HUMAN MILK

Feeding human milk is better tolerated, digested more quickly, stimulates the gastrointestinal system to grow, improves resistance to infection, and leads to better absorption of nutrients in the immature gut in comparison to formula. Bolstering the dose of mothers' milk an infant receives by 14 and 28 days of life has been shown to decrease the risk for sepsis by 19% for every 10 mL/kg/d of increase.[13] For each 10 mL/kg/d increase in human milk an infant receives during their NICU stay, a 0.35 increase in the cognitive index score is observed, and the overall dose of human milk an infant receives predicts survival.[14,15] Encouraging mothers to provide their human milk is cost effective, even though it requires concentrated and systematic effort across the health care team. One team showed that $534 in health care cost could be saved for every milliliter of milk provided in the first 14 days of life.[16] One health economist estimated that if the United States was to increase exposure to human milk for all preterm infants so that 90% of all preterm infants received 98% of their diet from human milk, $27 million in direct care costs and US$1.5 billion could be saved.[17] In fact, very conservative estimates indicate that optimizing exposure to human milk in the most fragile infants could translate to 928 fewer cases of NEC and also save 121 lives each year.[17]

ANTIINFLAMMATORY ROLE OF HUMAN MILK COMPONENTS

Human milk contains an estimate of thousands of bioactive components to provide specific nutrition for the infant.[18] Colostrum is the mothers' first milk and, although volumes are small compared with mature milk (as hormones to support lactation are increasing), this liquid gold provides higher levels of protein, triglycerides (fats), energy, and immune factors to the neonate.[19–21] As milk matures (postpartum day 5–11 average), components within the human milk change to best align for the continued support and protection of the neonate.[22] Human milk contains powerful immune support including antibodies from the mother (IgA), a free secretory component, lysozome, lactoferrin, lactoperoxidase, k-casein, haptocorrin, osteoprotegerin, and α-lactalbumin. Antioxidant factors work in the human body to decrease or eliminate free radicals, which decreases damage causing oxidative stress. In the neonate, oxidative stress can be caused by pain, organ damage, inflammation, oxygen toxicity, and other stressors common in the NICU and human milk is a powerful antioxidant.[23]

Cytokines within human milk are chemical mediators that play a major role in the inflammatory process. Classified as proinflammatory and antiinflammatory cytokines, they upregulate and downregulate the response to pathogens or tissue injury based on feedback processes. Chemokines are potent activators of neutrophils, which provide neonatal support of the infant's immune response to viral and bacterial pathogens.[10,23] Additionally, bioactive hormones and growth factors are human milk components that support the health and ongoing cell growth of the neonate. These include epidermal growth factors, transforming growth factor-α, transforming growth factor-β, and insulin-like growth factors, which are responsible for glucose control and metabolism; others support intestinal and systemic growth.[23]

Although each of these components plays a significant role in the protection and health of this at-risk population, several are described herein to highlight their immune function. Secretory IgA antibodies are considered to be one of the most important immunoglobulin isotypes found in both colostrum and mature milk. Providing an immunologic memory of the pathogens to which the mother has been exposed provides the infant with an essential rapid identification and reaction to pathogenic invasion.[15] Lactoferrin is a glycoprotein that has specific immunomodulation functions, specifically antimicrobial, antiinflammatory, and antioxidant properties. This glycoprotein is available in higher concentrations in preterm mother's milk.[24] Erythropoietin is the primary hormone responsible for red blood cell production. Preterm infants, especially those at risk for anemia, can benefit from this component of human milk. Anemia has been correlated with increased NEC risk in the preterm infant, and erythropoietin has effects on intestinal maturation that might be advantageous independent of replacing red cell volume.[25,26] Pluripotent stem cells are present in human milk.[27] These specific stem cells have the ability to differentiate into all 3 germ layers to repair and restore any cell in the body.[27] Regeneration of the intestinal lining via the actions of stem cells has been shown to be an important sign of a developing and functional intestinal mucosa that improves its barrier function.[28,29] Microbiota, including prebiotic and probiotic bacteria, are also present in breastmilk. These commensal bacteria include *Lactobacillus*, *Staphylococcus*, *Enterococcus*, and *Bifidobacterium*, offering protective colonization to the newborn gut.[30] Understanding the relationship between the gut microbiome alterations after maternal antibiotic use during delivery, mode of delivery, and postnatal antibiotic use highlights the importance of providing this method of establishing protective bacteria to the intestinal tract.

DISPARITIES IN HUMAN MILK USE

Despite evidence to support the health benefits of feeding human milk to fragile neonates, formula feeding is still common in NICUs within the United States. The frequency with which fragile neonates receive human milk at discharge is a quality metric tracked by every neonatal quality collaborative in the United States.[31–35] Rates of human milk feeding are shown to also vary across NICUs. In a 2008 analysis by Lake and colleagues,[32] 44% of US infants within the Vermont-Oxford Network were discharged home on any breastmilk, with marked differences among non-black (74%) compared with black infants (52%). Within the same network, estimated to include 558 of the 890 US NICUs,[32] rates of NEC also ranged from 6.9% in the lowest performing (ie, 90th percentile) to 3.7% in the highest performing (ie, 10th percentile).[36] It is possible that those NICUs who are not Vermont-Oxford Network members would report lower performance based on evidence that Vermont-Oxford Network centers are more often in teaching centers, have better nursing professional practice environments, be designated as magnet centers, and have lower nurse–patient ratios.[32]

In the United States, very low birth weight infants born to black mothers are significantly less likely to receive any human milk when compared with non-black infants (white and Hispanic).[37] In a study of 1034 extremely low birth weight infants (ELBW) weighing less than 1000 g cared for in 19 US NICUs, 64% of black infants received human milk compared with 84% of non-black infants.[38–40] Lake and colleagues[32] showed that disparities in exposure to human milk were particularly prevalent between NICUs serving predominantly white versus predominantly black families. When they evaluated the proportional racial composition of infants and the percentage of black infants discharged home on breastmilk, they showed that 24% of black infants in high black NICUs (>31%) received human milk compared with 41% in low black units (<11%) and that white infants also showed disparity based on their NICU of care.[32] Hallowell and colleagues[41] connected poor nursing work environments to lower exposures to human milk, which is important because promoting human milk feeding is a nursing-intense intervention. Just as nursing practice environments differ, the ratios of nurse–patient staffing differ, the support for human milk expression and expert lactation guidance is not consistent across NICUs.[37,42]

ENGAGING MOTHERS AND SUPPORTING BREASTFEEDING SELF-EFFICACY

Providing human milk to a fragile infant is an impossible task without engaging the mother in the process and educating parents about how human milk is a prevention measure for NEC. Social cognitive theory, with its emphasis on self-efficacy, is widely used to explain and predict maternal behaviors to initiate and continue breastfeeding.[43] Self-efficacy, the confidence or belief that one is able to do something, is a central determinant in behavior change.[44,45] One's beliefs about their ability (eg, to provide breast milk) has a causal influence on if they actually do it.[46,47] Feeding decisions requires informed parents who know the value of human milk, early initiation of pumping, consistent pumping, and adequate support.[48,49] Once a mother makes the decision to provide human milk, she needs support and encouragement from the staff and providers in the NICU to follow through and continue long-term pumping for her infant. In sum, to inspire action to provide human milk, the conversation should be focused on changing beliefs about human milk and should provide support to initiate and sustain milk supply.

Mothers inconsistently receive evidence-based education about the cost effectiveness and value of human milk as medicine to decrease their baby's risk of complications. NICU parents typically prefer to take an active role, but may not know how to do so.[50–52] In an international survey of parents whose infants had NEC (n = 110), 68% of parents were dissatisfied with the information they received about NEC before their infant was diagnosed, 73% reported receiving the information only as verbal instruction, and less than 5% reported that they were educated in a way that included print or technology-mediated materials. Among parent respondents, 44% of parents were not told about the value of breast milk.[53] Survey results demonstrated that parents wanted information earlier in the clinical course, using resources they could refer to later, and to be given ways to be a partner in their infant's care. In response to this study, our team has designed parent education resources in English and Spanish to facilitate conversations about NEC, emphasize prevention strategies and to teach parents NEC warning signs (available from https://www.neczero.nursing.arizona.edu/). By not presenting the message of milk as medicine, well-intentioned clinicians who do not wish to worry or burden parents are actually eliminating their choice to offer a life-saving intervention. Because initiation and maintenance of milk supply is a time-sensitive endeavor, a lack of willingness to promote breastfeeding self-efficacy early will result in missing the window of opportunity to do so.

LACTATION SUPPORT TO PROMOTE HUMAN MILK USE

Active and expert lactation support is needed for mothers to initiate and maintain goal milk supply, described as volumes exceeding 500 mL/d by 14 days after delivery.[13] Promoting early initiation (ie, by 6 hours after delivery and preferably within 2 hours) and consistency with pumping (ie, $\geq$8–10 times a day) is necessary to bring in and sustain adequate volumes for long-term success.[13] Yet the availability of lactation expertise, time for the bedside nurse to support early initiation and adequate pumping intensity, and consistency of messaging about the value of human milk impacts that success. Mothers also need access to the pump and supplies once they are sent home from the hospital, as well as supports to persist with pumping when separated from their hospitalized infant. This support can take the form of providing loaner pump programs to bridge access challenges over weekends, meal trays, advocating to the insurance company to pay for pumping supplies, and supporting quiet and private places to pump that are close to their infant's bedside. Making provisions for these supports allows the mother to provide fresh breast milk and to sustain pumping in the long term.

A major hurdle for pump-dependent mothers is "coming to volume" (goal $\geq$500 mL/d).[19] Daily pumped volume at week 1 or week 2 after birth predicts a mother's continuation of human milk feedings at discharge.[54,55] When mothers achieved volumes of 500 mL/d or greater by 14 days after birth, their likelihood to provide human milk at discharge was 3 times higher than if not.[54,55] This finding supports the importance of the NICU health care staff in providing consistent messaging to mothers to start early and pump often.

USE OF MOBILE HEALTH TO SUPPORT HUMAN MILK FEEDING

Although up to 87% of mothers in the NICU use smartphones and mobile devices to obtain health information—more often than books (56%) or brochures (33%)[56]—the evaluation of this technology to support NICU mothers is minimal. Davis and colleagues[57] reviewed 46 apps for parents and evaluated them using the Patient Education Materials Assessment Tool[58] for understandability and actionability. They found that most apps required linking to a website with more information, few (10%) were available in Spanish, and most did not link to source evidence. Most apps (70%) were understandable, but fewer than one-half were actionable.[57] Of the 46 apps, one addressed the needs of parents of premature infants, but none adequately captured breastmilk pumping, initiation, or sustainment of milk supply for mothers of fragile infants. A few new apps have been released to support breastfeeding recently. One example is the *Peekaboo ICU* parent support community's Preemie App, released in 2015. Led by Jodi and Mark Dalozell, the Peekaboo ICU parent community is one of the largest parent support communities. Their social networking sites have received more than 106,575 likes and 103,569 followers on Facebook, and 2067 likes on Twitter in addition to notable features on *The Today Show* and news outlets. The Preemie App is comprehensive, designed from the perspective of a NICU nurse who is active in caring for families and infants and trained as a lactation consultant. The app includes extensive information on nutrition in the NICU, including a pumping log, production over time graphs, and information about initiating and expressing human milk. More than 7000 individuals have downloaded the free no-advertising app and on average 200 users log in each day to use it. Clinicians can engage with parents by offering the app and helping them to use it to (1) make an informed decision to provide human milk, (2) initiate pumping within 6 hours of birth and preferably within 1 hour, (3) pumping at least 8 times a day, (4) tracking of goal volumes, and (5) following growth and the achievement of milestones over time. Although parents may find this app on their own, it is not widely known about or recommended by NICU clinicians. In short, finding ways to directly engage mothers in tracking their activities related to providing human milk will be an essential activity in coming years, but studies are needed to evaluate what effects it has on maternal and infant outcomes.

ROLE OF QUALITY IMPROVEMENT INITIATIVES TO OPTIMIZE HUMAN MILK FEEDING

Quality improvement initiatives, like those completed in California and Canada, reveal that systematically implementing practices to support human milk feeding over time lead to sustained reduction in NEC rates.[31,59] Alshaikh and colleagues[31] applied quality improvement methodology and tracked the use of mother's own milk (MOM) for preterm infants (<32 weeks gestation) before, during, and after the implementation of systematic practice changes to promote MOM use. The quality improvement intervention was composed of expanded access (within 6–12 hours after delivery) to and expertise of lactation consultants within the NICU to support early human milk expression and breast pump use; systematic education of mothers via handouts and multimedia content; widespread education of nurses about the value of and ways to support human milk; and use of tracking by the mother of volumes. In later quality improvement cycles, this team added earlier education about the value of human milk (ie, during the antepartum consultation), included more actively the postpartum nurses and lactation consultants, added lactation courses on the antepartum unit, and automatically generated the lactation referral within the standardized electronic order set for all infants born less than 32 weeks of gestation. Consequently, the rates of use of MOM at first feeding increased (from 61% to 74%; $P = .004$), the use of MOM when reaching 40 mL/kg/d increased (65% to 79%; $P<.001$), and the use of MOM at discharge improved (80% to 91%; $P<.001$). When confounders were addressed, the overall risk of NEC decreased between the baseline and sustain phase (odds ratio, 0.32; 95% confidence interval, 0.11–0.93), which represented a change from 8.9% to 4.7%.[31]

In California, Lee and colleagues[59] directed a human milk quality improvement project that recommended implementation of a change package to boost human milk use. Their lower baseline human milk exposure (54.6%) compared with the Canadian study improved significantly (to 61.7%; $P = .005$) and was sustained. As human milk exposure increased, NEC rates decreased (from 7.0% to 4.3%; $P = .022$). The change package included several elements, but the 3 focus areas addressed educating and advocating for MOM, strategies to establish and maintain maternal milk supply, and instituting a structured and consistent monitoring program for nutrition. When adjusting for multiple factors that may confound exposure, they found a 44% higher likelihood of breast milk feeding at discharge during the sustainability compared with baseline phases ($P<.05$). In short, as systematic improvements were made to increase human milk use the occurrence of NEC decreased (odds ratio, 0.36; 95% confidence interval, 0.17–0.76; $P<.05$).

Systematic integration of human milk promotion is a cornerstone of all effective quality improvement efforts to prevent and/or reduce NEC.[60–62] Although necessary, it may not be sufficient because other modifiable and nonmodifiable influences converge to create a perfect storm which ends in NEC. Recently, a multidisciplinary group called the NEC-Zero working group systematically and critically appraised the evidence for NEC prevention to arrive at a bundle of NEC prevention recommendations and implementation strategies. Core members of the team included parents of infants who got NEC, nurses, neonatal nurse practitioners, researchers, physicians, a dietitian, a pharmacist, and a lactation consultant. National partnerships with local experts to critique and define actionable implementation strategies that could be adopted immediately based on the balance of evidence quality, perceived benefit, and associated risk. Reported in a scoping review in 2017,[63] the core components promote (1) early and consistent promotion of human milk feeding beginning with colostrum for oral care, (2) unit-based adoption of a standardized feeding protocol, (3) stewardship of antibiotics and histamine-2 antagonists, and (4) a structured and consistent approach to risk recognition (ie, using a risk score like the GutCheck[NEC, 64] eNEC,[65] or NeoNEEDS[66]) and fostering structured communication between team members when NEC is suspected. Following the scoping review, an adherence score[67] and implementation checklist were developed to support consistent implementation of the bundle and to provide a clear way to audit and feed back to clinicians their progress. Clinical decision support technology to automate the bundle and to deploy the risk score for early warning were developed.

SUMMARY

NEC is a complex complication of prematurity. Multiple layers of protection, several of which are low cost and widely available, have been shown to be effective in the reduction of this neonatal morbidity. Understanding strategies to increase human milk use in the NICU, decrease racial and geographic disparities of human milk use, and a better understanding of human milk components are critical for the neonatal health care provider. Mothers are the keystone of quality improvement measures to decreasing NEC. Involving the parent early offering support for intention, initiation, maintenance, and sustaining of milk supply will require a comprehensive team approach. For NICU teams ready to implement change packages to promote the use of human milk, resources available from the California Perinatal Quality Collaborative[59] or NEC-Zero[63] could catalyze their work.

Best practices

What is the current practice for human milk and NEC?

- Providing human milk to fragile and very low birth weight infants is the standard of care.

- It is impossible to prevent NEC and provide human milk without including the mother as a critical partner in this process.

- Encouraging early and consistent exposure to human milk requires engaging the mother through early education about its benefits, availability of lactation support services, and comprehensive programs that provide consistent messaging about the value of human milk.

What changes in current practice are likely to improve outcomes?

- Antenatal consultation to share value of human milk is best when possible.

- Encouraging pumping by 2 hours after delivery, use of colostrum for oral care, tracking human milk volumes, assuring MOM is fed first, and deimplementing formula use until after 28 days of life has been shown to have the best protection against NEC.

ACKNOWLEDGMENTS

The authors thank the NEC-Zero working group for their work in 2015 to review evidence about human milk and to propose implementation strategies.

REFERENCES

1. Fanaroff AA, Stoll BJ, Wright LL, et al. Trends in neonatal morbidity and mortality for very low birthweight infants. Am J Obstet Gynecol 2007;196(2):147.e1-8.

2. Russell RB, Green NS, Steiner CA, et al. Cost of hospitalization for preterm and low birth weight infants in the United States. Pediatrics 2007;120(1):e1–9.

3. Schulman J, Stricof RL, Stevens TP, et al. Development of a statewide collaborative to decrease NICU central line-associated bloodstream infections. J Perinatol 2009;29(9):591–9.

4. Suresh GK, Edwards WH. Central line-associated bloodstream infections in neonatal intensive care: changing the mental model from inevitability to preventability. Am J Perinatol 2012;29(1):57–64.

5. Yee WH, Soraisham AS, Shah VS, et al. Incidence and timing of presentation of necrotizing enterocolitis in preterm infants. Pediatrics 2012;129(2):e298–304.

6. Pletsch D, Ulrich C, Angelini M, et al. Mothers' "liquid gold": a quality improvement initiative to support early colostrum delivery via oral immune therapy (OIT) to premature and critically ill newborns. Nurs Leadersh (Tor Ont) 2013; 26(Spec No 2013):34–42.

7. Cacho NT, Parker LA, Neu J. Necrotizing enterocolitis and human milk feeding: a systematic review. Clin Perinatol 2017;44(1):49–67.

8. Cortez J, Makker K, Kraemer DF, et al. Maternal milk feedings reduce sepsis, necrotizing enterocolitis and improve outcomes of premature infants. J Perinatol 2018;38(1):71–4.

9. Moore TA, Berger AM, Wilson ME. A new way of thinking about complications of prematurity. Biol Res Nurs 2014;16(1):72–82.

10. Ng PC, Li K, Wong RP, et al. Proinflammatory and anti-inflammatory cytokine responses in preterm infants with systemic infections. Arch Dis Child Fetal Neonatal Ed 2003;88(3):F209–13.

11. Garofalo R. Cytokines in human milk. J Pediatr 2010;156(2 Suppl):S36–40.

12. Moles L, Manzano S, Fernandez L, et al. Bacteriological, biochemical, and immunological properties of colostrum and mature milk from mothers of extremely preterm infants. J Pediatr Gastroenterol Nutr 2015;60(1):120–6.

13. Patel AL, Johnson TJ, Engstrom JL, et al. Impact of early human milk on sepsis and health-care costs in very low birth weight infants. J Perinatol 2013;33(7):514–9.

14. Patra K, Hamilton M, Johnson TJ, et al. NICU human milk dose and 20-month neurodevelopmental outcome in very low birth weight infants. Neonatology 2017;112(4):330–6.

15. Meinzen-Derr J, Poindexter B, Wrage L, et al. Role of human milk in extremely low birth weight infants' risk of necrotizing enterocolitis or death. J Perinatol 2009;29(1):57–62.

16. Johnson TJ, Patel AL, Bigger HR, et al. Cost savings of human milk as a strategy to reduce the incidence of necrotizing enterocolitis in very low birth weight infants. Neonatology 2015;107(4):271–6.

17. Colaizy TT, Bartick MC, Jegier BJ, et al. Impact of optimized breastfeeding on the costs of necrotizing enterocolitis in extremely low birthweight infants. J Pediatr 2016;175:100–5.e2.

18. Gidrewicz DA, Fenton TR. A systematic review and meta-analysis of the nutrient content of preterm and term breast milk. BMC Pediatr 2014;14:216.

19. Meier PP, Johnson TJ, Patel AL, et al. Evidence-based methods that promote human milk feeding of preterm infants: an expert review. Clin Perinatol 2017;44(1):1–22.

20. Zhang Y, Ji F, Hu X, et al. Oropharyngeal colostrum administration in very low birth weight infants: a randomized controlled trial. Pediatr Crit Care Med 2017;18(9):869–75.

21. Glass KM, Greecher CP, Doheny KK. Oropharyngeal administration of colostrum increases salivary secretory IgA levels in very low-birth-weight infants. Am J Perinatol 2017;34(14):1389–95.

22. Ballard O, Morrow AL. Human milk composition: nutrients and bioactive factors. Pediatr Clin North Am 2013;60(1):49–74.

23. Palmeira P, Carneiro-Sampaio M. Immunology of breast milk. Rev Assoc Med Bras (1992) 2016;62(6):584–93.

24. Manzoni P. Clinical benefits of lactoferrin for infants and children. J Pediatr 2016;173(Suppl):S43–52.

25. Patel RM, Knezevic A, Shenvi N, et al. Association of red blood cell transfusion, anemia, and necrotizing enterocolitis in very low-birth-weight infants. JAMA 2016;315(9):889–97.

26. Maheshwari A, Patel RM, Christensen RD. Anemia, red blood cell transfusions, and necrotizing enterocolitis. Semin Pediatr Surg 2018;27(1):47–51.

27. Briere CE, McGrath JM, Jensen T, et al. Breast milk stem cells: current science and implications for preterm infants. Adv Neonatal Care 2016;16(6):410–9.

28. Eaton S, Zani A, Pierro A, et al. Stem cells as a potential therapy for necrotizing enterocolitis. Expert Opin Biol Ther 2013;13(12):1683–9.

29. Zani A, Cananzi M, Fascetti-Leon F, et al. Amniotic fluid stem cells improve survival and enhance repair of damaged intestine in necrotising enterocolitis via a COX-2 dependent mechanism. Gut 2014;63(2):300–9.

30. Ramani M, Ambalavanan N. Feeding practices and necrotizing enterocolitis. Clin Perinatol 2013;40(1):1–10.

31. Alshaikh B, Kostecky L, Blachly N, et al. Effect of a quality improvement project to use exclusive mother's own milk on rate of necrotizing enterocolitis in preterm infants. Breastfeed Med 2015;10(7):355–61.

32. Lake ET, Staiger D, Horbar J, et al. Disparities in perinatal quality outcomes for very low birth weight infants in neonatal intensive care. Health Serv Res 2015; 50(2):374–97.

33. Parker MG, Burnham L, Mao W, et al. Implementation of a donor milk program is associated with greater consumption of mothers' own milk among VLBW infants in a US, level 3 NICU. J Hum Lact 2016;32(2):221–8.

34. Stone S, Lee HC, Sharek PJ. Perceived factors associated with sustained improvement following participation in a multicenter quality improvement collaborative. Jt Comm J Qual Patient Saf 2016;42(7):309–15.

35. Bixby C, Baker-Fox C, Deming C, et al. A multidisciplinary quality improvement approach increases breastmilk availability at discharge from the neonatal intensive care unit for the very-low-birth-weight infant. Breastfeed Med 2016;11(2): 75–9.

36. Horbar JD, Edwards EM, Greenberg LT, et al. Variation in performance of neonatal intensive care units in the United States. JAMA Pediatr 2017;171(3): e164396.

37. Boundy EO, Perrine CG, Nelson JM, et al. Disparities in hospital-reported breast milk use in neonatal intensive care units - United States, 2015. MMWR Morb Mortal Wkly Rep 2017;66(48):1313–7.

38. Vohr BR, Poindexter BB, Dusick AM, et al. Beneficial effects of breast milk in the neonatal intensive care unit on the developmental outcome of extremely low birth weight infants at 18 months of age. Pediatrics 2006;118(1):e115–23.

39. Fleurant E, Schoeny M, Hoban R, et al. Barriers to human milk feeding at discharge of very-low-birth-weight infants: maternal goal setting as a key social factor. Breastfeed Med 2017;12:20–7.

40. Sisk PM, Lovelady CA, Dillard RG, et al. Lactation counseling for mothers of very low birth weight infants: effect on maternal anxiety and infant intake of human milk. Pediatrics 2006;117(1):e67–75.

41. Hallowell SG, Rogowski JA, Spatz DL, et al. Factors associated with infant feeding of human milk at discharge from neonatal intensive care: cross-sectional analysis of nurse survey and infant outcomes data. Int J Nurs Stud 2016;53:190–203.

42. Engstrom JL, Patel AL, Meier PP. Eliminating disparities in mother's milk feeding in the neonatal intensive care unit. J Pediatr 2017;182:8–9.

43. Tuthill EL, McGrath JM, Graber M, et al. Breastfeeding self-efficacy: a critical review of available instruments. J Hum Lact 2016;32(1):35–45.

44. Bandura A, Wood R. Effect of perceived controllability and performance standards on self-regulation of complex decision making. J Pers Soc Psychol 1989; 56(5):805–14.

45. Bandura A. Self-Efficacy: the exercise of control. New York: W.H. Freeman; 1997.

46. Martinez-Brockman JL, Shebl FM, Harari N, et al. An assessment of the social cognitive predictors of exclusive breastfeeding behavior using the Health Action Process Approach. Soc Sci Med 2017;182:106–16.

47. Edwards ME, Jepson RG, McInnes RJ. Breastfeeding initiation: an in-depth qualitative analysis of the perspectives of women and midwives using Social Cognitive Theory. Midwifery 2018;57:8–17.

48. Richards CA, Starks H, O'Connor MR, et al. Elements of family-centered care in the pediatric intensive care unit: an integrative review. J Hosp Palliat Nurs 2017; 19(3):238–46.

49. Oliver S, Clarke-Jones L, Rees R, et al. Involving consumers in research and development agenda setting for the NHS: developing an evidence-based approach. Health Technol Assess 2004;8(15):1–148, iii–iv.

50. Partridge JC, Martinez AM, Nishida H, et al. International comparison of care for very low birth weight infants: parents' perceptions of counseling and decision-making. Pediatrics 2005;116(2):e263–71.

51. Tom DM, Aquino C, Arredondo AR, et al. Parent preferences for shared decision-making in acute versus chronic illness. Hosp Pediatr 2017;7(10):602–9.

52. Aronson PL, Shapiro ED, Niccolai LM, et al. Shared decision-making with parents of acutely ill children: a narrative review. Acad Pediatr 2018;18(1):3–7.

53. Gadepalli SK, Canvasser J, Eskenazi Y, et al. Roles and experiences of parents in necrotizing enterocolitis: an international survey of parental perspectives of communication in the NICU. Adv Neonatal Care 2017;17(6):489–98.

54. Meier PP, Engstrom JL, Mingolelli SS, et al. The Rush Mothers' Milk Club: breast-feeding interventions for mothers with very-low-birth-weight infants. J Obstet Gynecol Neonatal Nurs 2004;33(2):164–74.

55. Meier PP, Patel AL, Hoban R, et al. Which breast pump for which mother: an evidence-based approach to individualizing breast pump technology. J Perinatol 2016;36(7):493–9.

56. Orr T, Campbell-Yeo M, Benoit B, et al. Smartphone and internet preferences of parents: information needs and desired involvement in infant care and pain management in the NICU. Adv Neonatal Care 2017;17(2):131–8.

57. Davis DW, Logsdon MC, Vogt K, et al. Parent education is changing: a review of smartphone apps. MCN Am J Matern Child Nurs 2017;42(5):248–56.

58. Shoemaker SJ, Wolf MS, Brach C. Development of the Patient Education Materials Assessment Tool (PEMAT): a new measure of understandability and actionability for print and audiovisual patient information. Patient Educ Couns 2014; 96(3):395–403.

59. Lee HC, Kurtin PS, Wight NE, et al. A quality improvement project to increase breast milk use in very low birth weight infants. Pediatrics 2012;130(6):e1679–87.

60. Ellsbury DL, Clark RH, Ursprung R, et al. A multifaceted approach to improving outcomes in the NICU: the Pediatrix 100 000 Babies campaign. Pediatrics 2016;137(4) [pii:e20150389].

61. Talavera MM, Bixler G, Cozzi C, et al. Quality improvement initiative to reduce the necrotizing enterocolitis rate in premature infants. Pediatrics 2016;137(5) [pii: e20151119].

62. Patel AL, Panagos PG, Silvestri JM. Reducing incidence of necrotizing enterocolitis. Clin Perinatol 2017;44(3):683–700.

63. Gephart SM, Hanson C, Wetzel CM, et al. NEC-zero recommendations from scoping review of evidence to prevent and foster timely recognition of necrotizing enterocolitis. Matern Health Neonatol Perinatol 2017;3:23.

64. Gephart SM, Spitzer AR, Effken JA, et al. Discrimination of GutCheckNEC: a clinical risk index for necrotizing enterocolitis. J Perinatol 2014;34(6):468–75.

65. Naberhuis J, Wetzel C, Tappenden KA. A novel neonatal feeding intolerance and necrotizing enterocolitis risk-scoring tool is easy to use and valued by nursing staff. Adv Neonatal Care 2016;16(3):239–44.

66. Fox JR, Thacker LR, Hendricks-Muñoz KD. Early detection tool of intestinal dysfunction: impact on necrotizing enterocolitis severity. Am J Perinatol 2015; 32(10):927–32.

67. Gephart SM, Wyles C, Canvasser J. Expert consensus to weight an adherence score for audit and feedback of practices that prevent necrotizing enterocolitis in very low birth weight infants. Appl Nurs Res 2018;39:182–8.

Influence of Growth Factors on the Development of Necrotizing Enterocolitis

Rita D. Shelby, MD[a], Barrett Cromeens, DO[a],
Terrance M. Rager, MD[a], Gail E. Besner, MD[b],*

KEYWORDS

- Necrotizing enterocolitis • Growth factors • Intestinal injury

KEY POINTS

- Necrotizing enterocolitis (NEC) remains a significant health care problem in the premature infant.
- Growth factors have a significant role in the development and maintenance of the gastrointestinal tract.
- Select growth factors have been shown to protect the intestines in experimental models of NEC.
- Further investigation is required to elucidate the exact mechanisms and effects of these growth factors prior to their clinical use.

INTRODUCTION

Necrotizing enterocolitis (NEC) is the most frequent and most serious gastrointestinal (GI) surgical emergency in preterm infants.[1] Despite decades of research, it remains the leading cause of morbidity and mortality in neonates, occurring predominately in premature infants weighing less than 1500 g and those born before 36 weeks' gestation.[2] Advances in modern medical and clinical care have improved the survival of premature infants, yet the prevalence of NEC remains high. In the United States, approximately 12% of extremely premature infants, those weighing less than 1500 g, develop NEC, with up to 50% succumbing to the disease.[3] Severe NEC, characterized by full-thickness necrosis of the intestine with peritonitis and sepsis, occurs in up

Disclosure Statement: The authors report no proprietary or commercial interest in any product mentioned or concept discussed in this article.
[a] Department of Pediatric Surgery, Center for Perinatal Research, The Research Institute, Nationwide Children's Hospital, 700 Children's Drive, Columbus, OH 43205, USA; [b] Department of Pediatric Surgery, Nationwide Children's Hospital, FB6135, 700 Children's Drive, Columbus, OH 43205, USA
* Corresponding author.
E-mail address: Gail.Besner@NationwideChildrens.org

to 63% of NEC cases and requires life-saving surgical intervention.[2] Patients who survive and recover require prolonged care due to associated complications, including defects in growth and development, liver failure from prolonged use of total parental nutrition, and short bowel syndrome resulting in intestinal failure.[1] Epidemiologic studies have identified multiple complex factors associated with the development of NEC, with gut prematurity, formula feedings, and altered gut microbiome believed to have primary roles in disease pathogenesis.[1,4–6]

Growth factors play important roles in the health and development of the GI tract, with many involved in intestinal growth and repair from inflammation or injury.[7] It has been established that growth factors have critical effects on cellular proliferation, differentiation, and survival.[8] It is hypothesized that absence or reduced levels of specific growth factors normally present during gestation contribute to the development of NEC; however, this remains poorly understood. To date there have been various studies demonstrating altered levels of growth factors in injured tissues as well as changes in the response of injured tissue in the presence or absence of a given growth factor. Continued work toward understanding these factors and their roles may be of clinical value in the future prevention and treatment of NEC.

EPIDERMAL GROWTH FACTOR

Members of the epidermal growth factor (EGF) family are recognized as critical trophic factors for normal intestinal development.[9] Most EGF family members are first synthesized as transmembrane precursors, eventually undergoing proteolysis into the mature, secreted form of the growth factor. EGF family proteins have tyrosine kinase activity and activate the EGF receptor (EGFR), which has been identified predominantly on the basolateral surface of intestinal enterocytes.[9,10] EGF is a 53-amino-acid peptide with resistance to proteolytic degradation from the gastric pH normally encountered in the gastric lumen and GI tract.[11] The primary source of intestinal EGF is the submandibular salivary gland.[10] Human EGF expression remains poorly understood, with information on expression of salivary EGF and serum EGF levels in premature infants particularly lacking.[9]

Epidermal Growth Factor and the Intestine

Various studies have shown that EGF given in utero accelerates the maturation of intestinal enzyme activity and intestinal growth.[9] In addition, there is evidence that EGF stimulates intestinal growth. The importance of EGF has been demonstrated by the observation that EGFR knockout mice die prematurely or in utero.[12] Furthermore, mice that survive postnatally demonstrate significant epithelial underdevelopment in various tissues and develop severe hemorrhagic enteritis similar to human NEC.[9,13] EGF is present in various fluids that come into contact with the developing intestine, including amniotic fluid (AF), fetal urine, breast milk (BM), bile, and saliva.[9] In addition, EGF exerts potent trophic and cytoprotective effects on enterocytes, facilitating normal function, maturation, healing, and survival.[11,14] After intestinal mucosal injury, EGF promotes epithelial intestinal restitution, thus restoring gut barrier function and preventing bacterial translocation and resulting sepsis.[15,16] This is further enhanced by the ability of EGF to decrease apoptosis and moderate the proinflammatory response after injury.[17]

Epidermal Growth Factor and Necrotizing Enterocolitis

Various investigations have highlighted the importance of EGF in the pathogenesis and treatment of NEC. Immaturity of the developing gut leading to decreased intestinal mucosal barrier function, diminished restitution, impaired intestinal motility, and bacterial translocation are believed to contribute to NEC.[18–20] Premature infants have immature intestinal defenses and are often exposed to antibiotics and formula feedings that alter the intestinal microbiome. These factors are believed to increase pathogenic bacterial translocation.[21] Neonatal rat models have shown significantly decreased EGFR expression in the injured ilium of animals with NEC.[22] Furthermore, administration of EGF led to decreased incidence and severity of NEC through accelerated goblet cell maturation, mucin production, and normalization of enterocyte tight junction protein expression.[17] Although there are minimal human data, an association between EGF and human disease has been demonstrated.[23] Salivary EGF is significantly reduced in infants with NEC compared with premature infants who do not develop NEC,[9] with lower salivary EGF levels correlating with increasing prematurity.[24] Formula feeding is a well-known risk factor for NEC, one that can be mitigated to a degree with BM. BM and colostrum are the primary source of EGF postnatally, with EGF concentration inversely proportional to the gestational age of the infant.[25] Commercial infant formulas contain no EGF, which may explain why formula feeding in premature infants is considered a leading risk factor for the development of NEC.[25,26]

Epidermal Growth Factor and the Inflammatory Response

Another process believed to have significance in the pathogenesis of NEC is the altered inflammatory response, with a primarily proinflammatory cascade believed to have a major role.[25] In a neonatal rat model of NEC, elevated expression of proinflammatory cytokines interleukin (IL)-18 and IL-12 were directly associated with injury severity.[26] Furthermore, infants with NEC have high levels of proinflammatory platelet-activating factor, tumor necrosis factor α (TNF-α), IL-8, and nitric oxide (NO).[27] Enteral EGF administration results in decreased IL-18 and increased anti-inflammatory IL-10 expression during experimental NEC.[28]

Epidermal Growth Factor and Apoptosis

Another potential mechanism in the pathogenesis of NEC is enterocyte apoptosis. Apoptosis, mediated through BAX, is observed in rat models of NEC. It is believed to occur prior to the onset of fulminant disease and is influenced by EGF. EGF administration leads to decreased BAX and increased antiapoptotic Bcl-2 levels.[16]

Clinical Studies of Epidermal Growth Factor for Necrotizing Enterocolitis

Clinical studies of EGF as a treatment of NEC have been limited and have not provided much advance in its treatment or prevention. Further investigation is warranted, however, given that EGF has distinct roles in pathogenesis of experimental NEC.

HEPARIN-BINDING EPIDERMAL GROWTH FACTOR–LIKE GROWTH FACTOR

Heparin binding (HB)-EGF is a glycoprotein member of the EGF family, with expression triggered by hypoxia and oxidative stress. HB-EGF induces wound healing and tissue regeneration in response to tissue damage.[29] In addition to binding to the EGFR, HB-EGF binds and signals through a specific receptor, known as N-arginine dibasic convertase (NRDc), resulting in increased chemoattractant and migration activities.[30] It is believed that the EGFR-binding specificities of HB-EGF, along with its ability to signal though its specific NRDc receptor and its ability to bind to cell-surface heparin-sulfate proteoglycans, may combine to confer a particularly important functionality of HB-EGF compared with other members of the EGF family. HB-EGF is found in AF and BM, allowing its continuous exposure to fetal and newborn intestine.[31]

Endogenous HB-EGF is expressed in many cell types and is a potent mitogen for several of those cells, including cells of the intestinal mucosa.[32] Various animal models of intestinal injury have been used to demonstrate the effects of HB-EGF, with a significant amount of knowledge gained from work in the authors' laboratory.

Heparin-Binding Epidermal Growth Factor and Intestinal Restitution

Endogenous HB-EGF plays an important role in restitution.[33] Administration of HB-EGF activates the ErbB-1 receptor and subsequent signaling increases the rate of intestinal epithelial cell (IEC) migration, proliferation, and restitution after intestinal ischemia/reperfusion (I/R) injury[33] and experimental NEC.[34] HB-EGF also affects restitution by altering cell adhesion and by decreasing intercellular adhesion molecules.[35]

Heparin-Binding Epidermal Growth Factor and Intestinal Stem Cells

The intestinal epithelium is the most rapidly renewing tissue in mammals and is fueled by intestinal stem cells (ISCs) that reside at the base of the crypts. Intestinal injury of various forms damages not only differentiated IECs but also the ISCs required for restitution.[36] Enteral administration of HB-EGF protects ISCs and enterocytes from injury in experimental NEC.[37]

Heparin-Binding Epidermal Growth Factor and Mesenchymal Stem Cells

HB-EGF protects mesenchymal stem cells (MSCs) from hypoxia-induced apoptosis.[38] In models of NEC, intravenous and intraperitoneal administration of MSC protects the intestines from injury, with simultaneous administration of HB-EGF enhancing the beneficial effects of MSC.[39] HB-EGF likely not only protects injured ISCs but also preserves the viability of transplanted MSC, thus allowing these cells to play a greater role in intestinal healing.

Heparin-Binding Epidermal Growth Factor and the Enteric Nervous System

The premature GI tract has poor motility, likely from underdevelopment of the enteric nervous system (ENS), which is critical for coordinating peristalsis.[40] ENS abnormalities involving both neurons and glial cells exist in human intestine resected for NEC compared with age-matched intestine resected for non-NEC conditions.[41] HB-EGF has been shown to improve post-NEC intestinal motility by promotion of neural stem cell proliferation and migration.[42] Enteral administration of HB-EGF in rats exposed to NEC results in preservation of enteric neuronal NO synthase (NOS) levels with concomitant improvement in postinjury intestinal motility.[41]

Heparin-Binding Epidermal Growth Factor–Mediated Protection from Apoptosis

Apoptosis is triggered by the generation of reactive oxygen species (ROS) after oxidative stress, which is commonly seen in NEC. Apoptosis is believed to play either an etiologic role or to represent a final cellular pathway in the pathogenesis of NEC.[43] HB-EGF decreases IEC apoptosis after exposure to hypoxia in vitro[44] and reduces ROS production after enteral administration in a rat model of I/R injury.[45] Furthermore, HB-EGF decreases IEC apoptosis in a rat model of NEC.[46]

Heparin-Binding Epidermal Growth Factor and Inflammatory Mediators

Immune dysregulation is 1 potential etiologic factor associated with the development of NEC. In a rat model of I/R injury, HB-EGF administration decreased the serum levels of the proinflammatory cytokines TNF-α, IL-6, and IL-1β after injury.[47] During intestinal injury, inflammatory cytokines trigger an up-regulation of inducible NOS (iNOS), which generates large amounts of NO that is oxidized into reactive nitrogen species. Intraluminal administration of HB-EGF after intestinal I/R injury significantly decreases iNOS gene expression and protein production,[48] with subsequent decreased intestinal damage.

Heparin-Binding Epidermal Growth Factor and Gut Barrier Function

NEC is associated with decreased gut barrier function, increased intestinal permeability, and resultant bacterial translocation.[49] HB-EGF decreases bacterial translocation across IEC monolayers after I/R exposure.[50] In HB-EGF knockout mice, HB-EGF is shown essential for preservation of gut barrier function, in part due to inhibition of neutrophil-endothelial cell interactions.[51] In experimental models of NEC and other intestinal injury, exogenous enteral HB-EGF preserves gut barrier function.[48]

Heparin-Binding Epidermal Growth Factor and Human Necrotizing Enterocolitis

HB-EGF can protect the intestines from various forms of intestinal injury, including NEC. The beneficial effects observed in animal models may be applicable to humans. HB-EGF mRNA levels in human small bowel resected for NEC were higher at the resection margins adjacent to NEC-afflicted tissue, suggesting that lack of HB-EGF expression may play a role in the pathogenesis of NEC or that its expression may play a role in healing after injury.[5]

Clinical Studies of Heparin-Binding Epidermal Growth Factor for Human Necrotizing Enterocolitis

As of yet, there have been no clinical trials investigating the effects of HB-EGF in NEC. Until then, further investigations of HB-EGF in animal models will continue to elucidate the mechanisms by which this growth factor exerts its beneficial effects.

GLUCAGON-LIKE PEPTIDE 2

Glucagon-like peptide 2 (GLP-2) is an intestinotrophic hormone that is known for its proliferative and anti-inflammatory effects in the intestine. It is secreted from the L cells of the small and large intestine in response to fatty acids and glucose in the intestinal lumen and in response to ENS stimulation.[52] GLP-2 increases crypt cell proliferation, leading to increased villus height, crypt depth, and overall intestinal length.[53] There is incomplete knowledge of the downstream mechanisms of action of GLP-2, but animal models have shown promise in its ability to reduce the severity of NEC by maintaining the intestinal mucosa and reducing inflammatory cytokine production.[52]

Glucagon-Like Peptide 2 and Gut Development

GLP-2 signaling is hypothesized to play an important role in the developing intestine. The GLP-2 precursor, proglucagon, and the enzyme necessary for cleaving GLP-2 from proglucagon are found in rat fetal intestine, further supporting this theory.[54] Various studies have evaluated its effects and application in multiple GI diseases. GLP-2 administration results in increased intestinal growth and improved intestinal barrier function.[55] Animal studies demonstrate that it reduces histologic injury in experimental models of colitis.[56,57] Furthermore, there is increased mucosal villous height and proximal intestinal weight with exogenous GLP-2 administration in a premature piglet model of NEC.[55]

Glucagon-Like Peptide 2 and Inflammation

Multiple studies have demonstrated the anti-inflammatory effects of GLP-2 in the intestine. In a rat model of intestinal inflammation, GLP-2 administration led to reduced levels of the inflammatory cytokines interferon-λ, TNF-α, IL-1β, and iNOS.[58] In a rat model of NEC, GLP-2 administration resulted in decreased TNF-α and IL-6 levels that were comparable to dam-fed pups.[52] Finally, addition of GLP-2 to macrophages primed with lipopolysaccharides resulted in decreased proinflammatory iNOS, cyclooxygenase (COX)-2, TNF-α, IL-1β, and IL-6 levels.[58] Although knowledge of the exact mechanisms by which GLP-2 mediates its anti-inflammatory effects remains incomplete, there is continued study of its potential roles in inflammatory bowel disease.[59,60]

Glucagon-Like Peptide 2 and Necrotizing Enterocolitis

Several studies have demonstrated the ability of GLP-2 to attenuate intestinal injury.[61] There are few publications, however, on its role in NEC. A neonatal piglet model of NEC in which GLP-2 was administered demonstrated delayed onset of NEC from 10 hours to 25 hours; increased proximal jejunum weight, villous height, and area; and decreased histologic damage.[55] In this study, however, GLP-2 did not demonstrate a reduction in incidence of NEC or survival from NEC. Another study showed that high-dose GLP-2 administration in a rat model improved incidence and survival from NEC.[52] GLP-2 demonstrates potential in the treatment and prevention of NEC; however, additional investigation of its role is needed.

INSULIN-LIKE GROWTH FACTOR 1

Insulin-like growth factor-1 (IGF-1) is a polypeptide that is produced primarily in the liver. Circulating IGF-1 binds to the IGF-1 receptor (IGF-1R), leading to activation of intracellular signaling pathways that result in trophic effects on tissues.[62] IGF-1 is mainly present in BM and saliva. IGF-1R is present in the GI tract, with the highest concentration of the receptor found in the fetal GI tract.[63] IGF-1 promotes growth of the GI tract, participates in intestinal healing, and has anti-inflammatory properties, supporting research for IGF-1 as a possible treatment or prevention for NEC.[64]

Insulin-like Growth Factor 1 and Apoptosis

IGF-1 protects IECs from oxidative stress and apoptosis in the setting of intestinal injury.[65] It also promotes cytotoxic activity of natural killer cells.[66] In mouse and rat models of intestinal injury and experimental NEC, IGF-1 mitigated intestinal injury and decreased apoptosis.[67,68]

Insulin-like Growth Factor 1 and Gut Barrier Function

There is evidence suggesting that IGF-1 improves gut barrier function.[69] Furthermore, IGF-1 decreases bacterial translocation, likely due to its effect on gut barrier function.[70] When IGF-1 was administered in a rat model of small bowel transplantation, there was improvement in mucosal histology and enhanced gut barrier function.[71] In a human trial involving premature infants, formula supplemented with IGF-1 led to decreased gut permeability.[72] The anti-inflammatory effect of IGF-1 along with improved gut barrier function was demonstrated in a rat model of liver cirrhosis, where IGF-1 decreased intestinal mucosal damage and bacterial translocation, with up-regulation of anti-inflammatory COX-2 and down-regulation of TNF-α.[69]

Insulin-like Growth Factor 1 and Necrotizing Enterocolitis

Although limited, studies investigating the association of IGF-1 and NEC are promising. Early observations found that premature infants with persistently low IGF-1 levels had an increased risk of developing NEC.[7] Animal studies, using a mouse model of NEC, indicated that IGF-1 administration prior to injury resulted in decreased epithelial cell apoptosis and improved survival.[73]

Erythropoietin

Erythropoietin (EPO) is a glycoprotein secreted by the liver prenatally and by renal peritubular cells postnatally in response to anemia.[7] It is found in AF and BM, thereby providing access to its receptors in the developing GI tract, suggesting a potential role in the development, health, or proper function of the GI tract.[74,75] Animal models have demonstrated that EPO protects the GI tract by preservation of intestinal barrier function through tight junction protein expression[76] as well as protection against I/R injury.[77]

Erythropoietin in Experimental Intestinal Injury, Including Necrotizing Enterocolitis

Various animal studies have analyzed the mechanisms by which EPO affects different types of intestinal injury, including I/R injury, septic shock and hemorrhagic shock, inflammatory bowel disease, and NEC. In a rat model of intestinal I/R injury, a single dose of EPO decreased histologic injury and apoptosis and decreased markers of oxidative stress.[77] In a rat model of NEC, administration of EPO prior to injury resulted in decreased histologic injury and attenuated levels of NO, suggesting that EPO provides protection from oxidative damage in NEC.[78] EPO improves intestinal mucosal barrier integrity by regulating the expression of the tight junction protein zona occludens-1 (ZO-1) in a dose-dependent fashion.[76] Furthermore, administration of EPO in a rat model of NEC resulted in preservation of intestinal barrier function, decreased loss of ZO-1, and reduction in the incidence of NEC.[76]

Erythropoietin in Human Necrotizing Enterocolitis

Human studies of EPO in NEC are lacking. One retrospective cohort study of very-low-birthweight infants given recombinant EPO for prevention or treatment of anemia demonstrated a decreased incidence of NEC.[79] More recently, a randomized controlled trial of EPO in 90 premature infants showed that EPO improved feeding tolerance and decreased the risk of NEC.[80] Although there is potential for the use of EPO in treating and preventing NEC, further investigation is necessary.

GROWTH HORMONE

Growth hormone (GH) is a protein produced by the anterior pituitary gland with systemic effects on anabolism. GH reacts with its receptor, GH receptor, a transmembrane tyrosine kinase receptor, which is present in the GI tract. Upon binding to GH receptor, transcription of various genes occurs, resulting in glucose and lipid metabolic changes.[81] GH has an effect on the release and function of downstream intestinotrophic mediators, such as IGF-1, that have been implicated in the development of NEC.

GH is predominantly known for its impact on growth throughout the body. Short stature results from GH deficiency whereas gigantism and acromegaly result from GH excess. When introduced into the intestine, GH induces cell proliferation, decreased apoptosis, and preserves gut barrier function.[81] Additionally, recombinant human GH administration to rats with GH deficiency results in increased growth of each layer of the colonic wall.[82] There is ongoing investigation in the potential use of GH as a treatment or prevention of intestinal injury. Further studies to establish the role of GH in NEC are needed.

HEPATOCYTE GROWTH FACTOR

Hepatocyte growth factor (HGF) is a glycoprotein involved in angiogenesis, cellular proliferation, and survival.[7] Active HGF is found in the fetal GI tract as well as in BM and is involved in epithelial migration, proliferation, and repair of injured tissues.[83] Once activated, HGF binds to tyrosine kinase receptors with downstream effects on cell proliferation, apoptosis, and immunity regulation.[84] HGF is vital for embryonic development, as shown in a study where HGF deficient mice experience embryonic demise.[85] The mechanisms by which HGF exerts its effects are incompletely understood; thus, further research is required.

HGF has been shown to protect and repair intestinal tissue in many animal models. When given prior to I/R injury in rats, there was decreased apoptotic activity in the intestinal epithelium.[86] Mice with HGF receptor deficiency that were exposed to dextran sulfate sodium–induced or acetic acid–induced colitis had impaired colonic mucosal regeneration and increased mortality.[87] Finally, administration of enteral HGF decreased the incidence and severity of NEC in rats.[88]

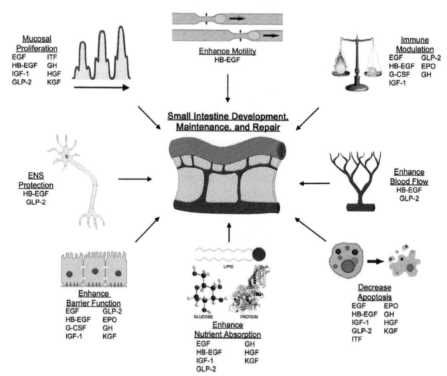

Fig. 1. Growth factors contribute to the development, maintenance, and repair of the small intestine. Research has led to the discovery of their roles in mucosal proliferation, enhancing motility, immune modulation, enhanced blood flow, decreased apoptosis, enhanced nutrient absorption, enhanced barrier function, and ENS protection. The growth factors are listed according to their proposed general mechanisms. G-CSF, granulocyte colony stimulating factor; ITF, intestinal trefoil factor; KGF, keratinocyte growth factor.

OTHER GROWTH FACTORS IN NECROTIZING ENTEROCOLITIS

The information presented in this article is a snapshot of the knowledge that is gained daily about a multitude of growth factors and their roles in the development and treatment of NEC. There are other growth factors that remain under investigation that were not included in this article. These include keratinocyte growth factor, intestinal trefoil factor, and granulocyte colony-stimulating factor, which have been identified as having a role in NEC. These additional growth factors have been associated with stimulation of mucosal proliferation, reducing apoptosis, modulating the immune system, and enhancing gut barrier function and nutrient absorption.[89–91]

SUMMARY

Growth factors play an important role in the development, growth, and health of the GI tract (**Fig. 1**). Through mediation of cellular activities, they have a role in cellular proliferation, migration, differentiation, and survival. Growth factors are present in AF and BM, thus having the potential to bathe intestinal cells, prenatally and postnatally. A relationship has been established between the presence of growth factors and disease severity, and healing potential in intestinal injury has been observed. For each of the growth factors reviewed in this article, and many others not reviewed, the current body of research is varied and evolving. Some, like EGF and HB-EGF, have been a significant focus of research related to NEC, whereas others are only recently beginning to be reported. Additional studies are needed to further elucidate the roles of these growth factors in the pathogenesis of NEC. Eventually, growth factors may lead to the development of novel therapies for the prevention and/or treatment of clinical NEC.

REFERENCES

1. Hunter CJ, Upperman JS, Ford HR, et al. Understanding the susceptibility of the premature infant to necrotizing enterocolitis (NEC). Pediatr Res 2008;63(2): 117–23.
2. Lee JS, Polin RA. Treatment and prevention of necrotizing enterocolitis. Semin Neonatol 2003;8(6):449–59.
3. Gephart SM, McGrath JM, Effken JA, et al. Necrotizing enterocolitis risk: state of the science. Adv Neonatal Care 2012;12(2):77–89.
4. Caplan MS, Jilling T. Neonatal necrotizing enterocolitis: possible role of probiotic supplementation. J Pediatr Gastroenterol Nutr 2000;30(Suppl 2):S18–22.
5. Feng J, El-Assal ON, Besner GE. Heparin-binding EGF-like growth factor (HB-EGF) and necrotizing enterocolitis. Semin Pediatr Surg 2005;14(3):167–74.
6. Schwiertz A, Gruhl B, Löbnitz M, et al. Development of the intestinal bacterial composition in hospitalized preterm infants in comparison with breast-fed, full-term infants. Pediatr Res 2003;54(3):393–9.
7. Rowland KJ, Choi PM, Warner BW. The role of growth factors in intestinal regeneration and repair in necrotizing enterocolitis. Semin Pediatr Surg 2013;22(2): 101–11.
8. McMellen ME, Wakeman D, Longshore SW, et al. Growth factors: possible roles for clinical management of the short bowel syndrome. Semin Pediatr Surg 2010; 19:35–43.
9. Warner BW, Warner BB. Role of epidermal growth factor in the pathogenesis of neonatal necrotizing enterocolitis. Semin Pediatr Surg 2005;14:175–80.

10. Playford RJ, Hanby AM, Gschmeissner S, et al. The epidermal growth factor receptor (EGF-R) is present on the basolateral, but not the apical, surface of enterocytes in the human gastrointestinal tract. Gut 1996;39(2):262–6.

11. Britton JR, George-Nascimento C, Udall JN, et al. Minimal hydrolysis of epidermal growth factor by gastric fluid of preterm infants. Gut 1989;30(3):327–32.

12. Li AK, Schattenkerk ME, Huffman RG, et al. Hypersecretion of submandibular saliva in male mice: trophic response in small intestine. Gastroenterology 1983; 84(5 Pt 1):949–55.

13. Miettinen PJ, Berger JE, Meneses J, et al. Epithelial immaturity and multiorgan failure in mice lacking epidermal growth factor receptor. Nature 1995; 376(6538):337–41.

14. Clark JA, Doelle SM, Halpern MD, et al. Intestinal barrier failure during experimental necrotizing enterocolitis: protective effect of EGF treatment. Am J Physiol Gastrointest Liver Physiol 2006;291(5):G938–49.

15. Miller CA, Debas HT. Epidermal growth factor stimulates the restitution of rat gastric mucosa in vitro. Exp Physiol 1995;80(6):1009–18.

16. Wilson AJ, Gibson PR. Role of epidermal growth factor receptor in basal and stimulated colonic epithelia cell migration in vitro. Exp Cell Res 1999;250:187–96.

17. Clark JA, Lane RH, Maclennan NK, et al. Epidermal growth factor reduces intestinal apoptosis in an experimental model of necrotizing enterocolitis. Am J Physiol Gastrointest Liver Physiol 2005;288(4):G755–62.

18. Berseth CL. Gut motility and the pathogenesis of necrotizing enterocolitis. Clin Perinatol 1994;21:263–70.

19. Halpern MD, Denning PW. The role of intestinal epithelial barrier function in the development of NEC. Tissue Barriers 2015;3(1–2):e1000707.

20. Claud EC, Walker WA. Hypothesis: inappropriate colonization of the premature intestine can cause neonatal necrotizing enterocolitis. FASEB J 2001;15(8): 1398–403.

21. Hodzic Z, Bolock AM, Good M. The role of mucosal immunity in the pathogenesis of necrotizing enterocolitis. Front Pediatr 2017;5:40.

22. Dvorak B, Halpern MD, Holubee H, et al. Epidermal growth factor reduces the development of necrotizing enterocolitis in a neonatal rat model. Am J Physiol Gastrointest Liver Physiol 2002;282:G156–64.

23. Shin CE, Falcone RA Jr, Stuart L, et al. Diminished epidermal growth factor levels in infants with necrotizing enterocolitis. J Pediatr Surg 2000;35:173–6.

24. Warner BB, Ryan AL, Seeger KJ, et al. Ontogeny of salivary epidermal growth factor and necrotizing enterocolitis. J Pediatr 2007;150:358–63.

25. Dvorak B, Fituch CC, Williams CS, et al. Concentrations of epidermal growth factor and transforming growth factor-alpha in preterm milk. Adv Exp Med Biol 2004; 554:407–9.

26. Xiao X, Xiong A, Chen X, et al. Epidermal growth factor concentrations in human milk, cow's milk and cow's milk-based infant formulas. Chin Med J (Engl) 2002; 115(3):451–4.

27. Caplan MS, Simon D, Jilling T. The role of PAF, TLR, and the inflammatory response in neonatal necrotizing enterocolitis. Semin Pediatr Surg 2005;14(3): 145–51.

28. Halpern MD, Dominguez JA, Dvorakova K, et al. Ileal cytokine dysregulation in experimental necrotizing enterocolitis is reduced by epidermal growth factor. J Pediatr Gastroenterol Nutr 2003;36(1):126–33.

29. Jin K, Mao XO, Sun Y, et al. Heparin-binding epidermal growth factor-like growth factor: hypoxia-inducible expression in vitro and stimulation of neurogenesis in vitro and in vivo. J Neurosci 2002;22(13):5365–73.
30. Nishi E, Prat A, Hospital V, et al. N-arginine dibasic convertase is a specific receptor for heparin-binding EGF-like growth factor that mediates cell migration. EMBO J 2001;20(13):3342–50.
31. Michalsky MP, Lara-Marquez M, Chun L, et al. Heparin-binding EGF-like growth factor is present in human amniotic fluid and breast milk. J Pediatr Surg 2002; 37(1):1–6.
32. Davis-Fleischer KM, Besner GE. Structure and function of heparin-binding EGF-like growth factor (HB-EGF). Front Biosci 1998;3:288–99.
33. El-Assal ON, Besner GE. HB-EGF enhances restitution after intestinal ischemia/reperfusion via PI3K/Akt and MEK/ERK1/2 activation. Gastroenterology 2005; 129(2):609–25.
34. Feng J, Besner GE. Heparin-binding epidermal growth factor-like growth factor promotes enterocyte migration and proliferation in neonatal rats with necrotizing enterocolitis. J Pediatr Surg 2007;42(1):214–20.
35. Su Y, Yang J, Besner GE. HB-EGF promotes intestinal restitution by affecting integrin-extracellular matrix interactions and intercellular adhesions. Growth Factors 2013;31(1):39–55.
36. Markel TA, Crisostomo PR, Lahm T, et al. Stem cells as a potential future treatment of pediatric intestinal disorders. J Pediatr Surg 2008;43(11):1953–63.
37. Chen CL, Yu X, James IO, et al. Heparin-binding EGF-like growth factor protects intestinal stem cells from injury in a rat model of necrotizing enterocolitis. Lab Invest 2012;92(3):331–44.
38. Watkins DJ, Zhou Y, Chen CL, et al. Heparin-binding epidermal growth factor-like growth factor protects mesenchymal stem cells. J Surg Res 2012;177(2):359–64.
39. Yang J, Watkins D, Chen CL, et al. Heparin-binding epidermal growth factor-like growth factor and mesenchymal stem cells act synergistically to prevent experimental necrotizing enterocolitis. J Am Coll Surg 2012;215(4):534–45.
40. Barlow AJ, Wallace AS, Thapar N, et al. Critical numbers of neural crest cells are required in the pathways from the neural tube to the foregut to ensure complete enteric nervous system formation. Development 2008;135(9):1681–91.
41. Zhou Y, Yang J, Watkins DJ, et al. Enteric nervous system abnormalities are present in human necrotizing enterocolitis: potential neurotransplantation therapy. Stem Cell Res Ther 2013;4(6):157.
42. Wei J, Zhou Y, Besner GE. Heparin-Binding EGF-like growth factor and enteric neural stem cell transplantation in the prevention of experimental necrotizing enterocolitis. Pediatr Res 2015;78(1):29–37.
43. Kim M, Christley S, Alverdy JC, et al. Immature oxidative stress management as a unifying principle in the pathogenesis of necrotizing enterocolitis: insights from an agent-based model. Surg Infect (Larchmt) 2012;13(1):8–32.
44. Michalsky MP, Kuhn A, Mehta V, et al. Heparin-binding EGF-like growth factor decreases apoptosis in intestinal epithelial cells in vitro. J Pediatr Surg 2001;36(8): 130–5.
45. Kuhn MA, Xia G, Mehta VB, et al. Heparin-binding EGF-like growth factor (HB-EGF) decreases oxygen free radical production in vitro and in vivo. Antioxid Redox Signal 2002;4(4):639–46.
46. Feng J, El-Assal ON, Besner GE. Heparin-binding epidermal growth factor-like growth factor reduces intestinal apoptosis in neonatal rats with necrotizing enterocolitis. J Pediatr Surg 2006;41(4):742–7.

47. Rocourt DV, Mehta VB, Besner GE. Heparin-binding EGF-like growth factor decreases inflammatory cytokine expression after intestinal ischemia/reperfusion injury. J Surg Res 2007;139(2):269–73.

48. Xia G, Lara-Marquez M, Luquette MH, et al. Heparin-binding EGF-like growth factor decreases inducible nitric oxide synthase and nitric oxide production after intestinal ischemia/reperfusion injury. Antioxid Redox Signal 2001;3(5):919–30.

49. Anand RJ, Leaphart CL, Mollen KP, et al. The role of the intestinal barrier in the pathogenesis of necrotizing enterocolitis. Shock 2007;27(2):124–33.

50. Xia G, Martin AE, Michalsky MP, et al. Heparin-binding EGF-like growth factor preserves crypt cell proliferation and decreases bacterial translocation after intestinal ischemia/reperfusion injury. J Pediatr Surg 2002;37(7):1081–7.

51. Zhang HY, Radulescu A, Besner GE. Heparin-binding epidermal growth factor-like growth factor is essential for preservation of gut barrier function after hemorrhagic shock and resuscitation in mice. Surgery 2009;146(2):334–9.

52. Nakame K, Kaji T, Mukai M, et al. The protective and anti-inflammatory effects of glucagon-like peptide-2 in an experimental rat model for necrotizing enterocolitis. Peptides 2016;75:1–7.

53. Rowland KJ, Brubaker PL. The "cryptic" mechanism of action of glucagon-like peptide-2. Am J Physiol Gastrointest Liver Physiol 2011;301(1):G1–8.

54. Lee YC, Brubaker PL, Drucker DJ. Developmental and tissue-specific regulation of proglucagon gene expression. Endocrinology 1990;127(5):2217–22.

55. Benight NM, Stoll B, Olutoye OO, et al. GLP-2 delays but does not prevent the onset of necrotizing enterocolitis in preterm pigs. J Pediatr Gastroenterol Nutr 2013;56(6):623–30.

56. Alavi K, Schwartz MZ, Palazzo JP, et al. Treatment of inflammatory bowel disease in a rodent model with the intestinal growth factor glucagon-like peptide-2. J Pediatr Surg 2000;35:847–51.

57. Yazbeck R, Sulda ML, Howarth GS, et al. Dipeptidyl peptidase expression during experimental colitis in mice. Inflamm Bowel Dis 2010;16:1340–51.

58. Xie S, Liu B, Fu S, et al. GLP-2 suppresses LPS-induced inflammation in macrophages by inhibiting ERK phosphorylation and NF-kappaB activation. Cell Physiol Biochem 2014;34(2):590–602.

59. Sigalet DL, Kravarusic D, Butzner D, et al. A pilot study examining the relationship among Crohn disease activity, glucagon-like peptide-2 signalling and intestinal function in pediatric patients. Can J Gastroenterol 2013;27(10):587–92.

60. Blonski W, Buchner AM, Aberra F, et al. Teduglutide in Crohn's disease. Expert Opin Biol Ther 2013;13(8):1207–14.

61. Drucker DJ, Yusta B, Boushey RP, et al. Human [Gly2]GLP-2 reduces the severity of colonic injury in a murine model of experimental colitis. Am J Physiol 1999; 276(1 Pt 1):G79–91.

62. Latres E, Amini AR, Amini AA, et al. Insulin-like growth factor-1 (IGF-1) inversely regulates atrophy-induced genes via the phosphatidylinositol 3-kinase/Akt/mammalian target of rapamycin (PI3K/Akt/mTOR) pathway. J Biol Chem 2005; 280(4):2737–44.

63. Freier S, Eran M, Reinus C, et al. Relative expression and localization of the insulin-like growth factor system components in the fetal, child and adult intestine. J Pediatr Gastroenterol Nutr 2005;40(2):202–9.

64. Tian F, Liu GR, Li N, et al. Insulin-like growth factor I reduces the occurrence of necrotizing enterocolitis by reducing inflammatory response and protecting intestinal mucosal barrier in neonatal rat model. Eur Rev Med Pharmacol Sci 2017; 21(20):4711–9.

65. Wilkins HR, Ohneda K, Keku TO, et al. Reduction of spontaneous and irradiation-induced apoptosis in small intestine of IGF-I transgenic mice. Am J Physiol Gastrointest Liver Physiol 2002;283(2):G457–64.

66. Ni F, Sun R, Fu B, et al. IGF-1 promotes the development and cytotoix activity of human NK cells. Nat Commun 2013;4:1479.

67. Jeschke MG, Bolder U, Chung DH, et al. Gut mucosal homeostasis and cellular mediators after severe thermal trauma and the effect of insulin-like growth factor-I in combination with insulin-like growth factor binding protein-3. Endocrinology 2007;148(1):354–62.

68. Ozen S, Akisu M, Baka M, et al. Insulin-like growth factor attenuates apoptosis and mucosal damage in hypoxia/reoxygenation-induced intestinal injury. Biol Neonate 2005;87(2):91–6.

69. Lorenzo-Zuniga V, Rodríguez-Ortigosa CM, Bartolí R, et al. Insulin-like growth factor I improves intestinal barrier function in cirrhotic rats. Gut 2006;55(9):1306–12.

70. Hunninghake GW, Doerschug KC, Nymon AB, et al. Insulin-like growth factor-1 levels contribute to the development of bacterial translocation in sepsis. Am J Respir Crit Care Med 2010;182(4):517–25.

71. Zhang W, Frankel WL, Adamson WT, et al. Insulin-like growth factor-I improves mucosal structure and function in transplanted rat small intestine. Transplantation 1995;59(5):755–61.

72. Corpeleijn WE, van Vliet I, de Gast-Bakker DA, et al. Effect of enteral IGF-1 supplementation on feeding tolerance, growth, and gut permeability in enterally fed premature neonates. J Pediatr Gastroenterol Nutr 2008;46(2):184–90.

73. Baregamian N, Rychahou PG, Hawkins HK, et al. Phosphatidylinositol 3-kinase pathway regulates hypoxia-inducible factor-1 to protect from intestinal injury during necrotizing enterocolitis. Surgery 2007;142(2):295–302.

74. Juul SE, Zhao Y, Dame JB, et al. Origin and fate of erythropoietin in human milk. Pediatr Res 2000;48(5):660–7.

75. Yu Y, Shiou S-R, Guo Y, et al. Erythropoietin protects epithelial cells from excessive autophagy and apoptosis in experimental neonatal necrotizing enterocolitis. PLoS One 2013;8(7):e69620.

76. Shiou SR, Yu Y, Chen S, et al. Erythropoietin protects intestinal epithelial barrier function and lowers the incidence of experimental neonatal necrotizing enterocolitis. J Biol Chem 2011;286(14):12123–32.

77. Guneli E, Cavdar Z, Islekel H, et al. Erythropoietin protects the intestine against ischemia/reperfusion injury in rats. Mol Med 2007;13(9–10):509–17.

78. Kumral A, Baskin H, Duman N, et al. Erythropoietin protects against necrotizing enterocolitis of newborn rats by the inhibiting nitric oxide formation. Biol Neonate 2003;84(4):325–9.

79. Ledbetter DJ, Juul SE. Erythropoietin and the incidence of necrotizing enterocolitis in infants with very low birth weight. J Pediatr Surg 2000;35(2):178–81.

80. El-Ganzoury MM, Awad HA, El-Farrash RA, et al. Enteral granulocyte-colony stimulating factor and erythropoietin early in life improves feeding tolerance in preterm infants: a randomized controlled trial. J Pediatr 2014;165(6):1140–5.e1.

81. Rosenfeld RG, Hwa V. The growth hormone cascade and its role in mammalian growth. Horm Res 2009;71(Suppl 2):36–40.

82. Tei TM, Kissmeyer-Nielsen P, Christensen H, et al. Growth hormone treatment increases transmural colonic growth in GH-deficient dwarf rats. Growth Horm IGF Res 2000;10(2):85–92.

83. Ido A, Numata M, Kodama M, et al. Mucosal repair and growth factors: recombinant human hepatocyte growth factor as an innovative therapy for inflammatory bowel disease. J Gastroenterol 2005;40(10):925–31.
84. Zarnegar R, Michalopoulos GK. The many faces of hepatocyte growth factor: from hepatopoiesis to hematopoiesis. J Cell Biol 1995;129(5):1177–80.
85. Uehara Y, Minowa O, Mori C, et al. Placental defect and embryonic lethality in mice lacking hepatocyte growth factor/scatter factor. Nature 1995;373(6516): 702–5.
86. Kuenzler KA, Pearson PY, Schwartz MZ. Hepatocyte growth factor pretreatment reduces apoptosis and mucosal damage after intestinal ischemia-reperfusion. J Pediatr Surg 2002;37(7):1093–7.
87. Itoh H, Naganuma S, Takeda N, et al. Regeneration of injured intestinal mucosa is impaired in hepatocyte growth factor activator-deficient mice. Gastroenterology 2004;127(5):1423–35.
88. Jain SK, Baggerman EW, Mohankumar K, et al. Amniotic fluid-borne hepatocyte growth factor protects rat pups against experimental necrotizing enterocolitis. Am J Physiol Gastrointest Liver Physiol 2014;306(5):G361–9.
89. Cai Y, Wang W, Liang H, et al. Keratinocyte growth factor pretreatment prevents radiation-induced intestinal damage in a mouse model. Scand J Gastroenterol 2013;48(4):419–26.
90. Taupin DR, Kinoshita K, Podolsky DK. Intestinal trefoil factor confers colonic epithelial resistance to apoptosis. Proc Natl Acad Sci U S A 2000;97(2):799–804.
91. MohanKumar K, Kaza N, Jagadeeswaran R, et al. Gut mucosal injury in neonates is marked by macrophage infiltration in contrast to pleomorphic infiltrates in adult: evidence from an animal model. Am J Physiol Gastrointest Liver Physiol 2012; 303(1):G93–102.

Can Fish Oil Reduce the Incidence of Necrotizing Enterocolitis by Altering the Inflammatory Response?

Brandy L. Frost, MD*, Michael S. Caplan, MD

KEYWORDS

- Necrotizing enterocolitis • Prematurity • Very low birth weight • Fish oil
- Omega-3 long-chain polyunsaturated fatty acids

KEY POINTS

- Despite modern advances in neonatology, necrotizing enterocolitis continues to affect preterm infants, particularly very low-birth-weight infants.
- Necrotizing enterocolitis is characterized by a robust inflammatory response.
- Fish oil, containing docosahexaenoic acid and eicosapentaenoic acid, exerts anti-inflammatory effects via multiple mechanisms of action.
- Previous animal and human studies have demonstrated the potential for fish oil to modulate inflammation; thus, fish oil supplementation may be able to reduce necrotizing enterocolitis incidence.

INTRODUCTION

The final trimester of pregnancy is a time of significant nutritional and metabolic changes for the fetus. With regards to long-chain polyunsaturated fatty acids (LCPUFA), the greatest accretion occurs in the third trimester, a time of rapid growth as well as of development of the brain. As such, infants who are born prematurely do not benefit from this in utero support. Furthermore, after birth, the smallest and sickest preterm infants are often dependent on a parenteral supply of nutrition, and many intravenous lipid preparations in the neonatal intensive care unit (NICU) are devoid of LCPUFA. Although LCPUFA-supplemented enteral feedings are slowly advanced,

Disclosures: Dr B.L. Frost receives research support from Mead Johnson Nutrition and Leadiant Biosciences, and Dr M.S. Caplan is a paid speaker for Mead Johnson Nutrition as well as a consultant for Leadiant Biosciences.
Department of Pediatrics, NorthShore University HealthSystem, University of Chicago Pritzker School of Medicine, 2650 Ridge Avenue, Walgreen Building Suite 1505, Evanston, IL 60201, USA
* Corresponding author.
E-mail address: bfrost@northshore.org

Clin Perinatol 46 (2019) 65–75
https://doi.org/10.1016/j.clp.2018.09.004
0095-5108/19/© 2018 Elsevier Inc. All rights reserved.

the preterm infant quickly becomes deficient in these important fatty acids. The authors and others have shown that LCPUFA levels drop within 2 weeks of birth,[1] and therefore, preterm infants are quite deficient in LCPUFA compared with normal in utero accretion.

Previous studies demonstrate a benefit for newborns from LCPUFA with respect to brain and eye development,[2–6] in both term and preterm infants, such that LCPUFA supplementation is now standard of care in term and preterm formula. Furthermore, docosahexaenoic acid (DHA) is the main lipid in the central nervous system. There are varying levels of LCPUFA in breast milk, depending on maternal diet.[7]

In addition to the benefits shown on eye and brain development, LCPUFA have been shown to modulate the inflammatory cascade. In vitro studies demonstrate anti-inflammatory effects via several mechanisms, and both animal and human data support an anti-inflammatory role, particularly for the omega-3 LCPUFAs, such as DHA. Recent studies have focused on the interaction between LCPUFA levels and bronchopulmonary dysplasia (BPD),[8] but it is plausible that supplementation with LCPUFA may also modify risk for other neonatal morbidities, such as sepsis and necrotizing enterocolitis (NEC). In this review, the authors examine the evidence to support a role for LCPUFA in modulating the risk for NEC.

Necrotizing Enterocolitis

NEC is a devastating inflammatory bowel necrosis affecting predominantly preterm infants. This disease affects approximately 10% of infants born weighing less than 1500 g, although the incidence varies widely in published studies as well as by center and region. Several risk factors for NEC are well described, including prematurity, formula feeding, intestinal ischemia, and bacterial colonization. Current dogma supports a theory of an imbalance between proinflammatory and anti-inflammatory forces in the preterm infant, with a shift toward a proinflammatory state in the preterm infant as compared with full-term infants.

As such, preventative strategies to shift the balance toward a more anti-inflammatory profile may show promise in reducing NEC risk. Because NEC often presents very acutely and is even fulminant in certain cases, the focus is on prevention rather than treatment. Once diagnosed, the treatment is largely supportive, rather than specific. Human and animal studies have examined the preventative role of probiotics,[9–11] lactoferrin,[12] erythropoietin,[13] and growth factors.[14,15] Because of their anti-inflammatory mechanism of action, LCPUFA, and in particular, the omega-3 LCPUFA, are an intriguing potential preventative measure.

Long-Chain Polyunsaturated Fatty Acids and Inflammation

With regards to LCPUFA, the omega-3 fatty acids eicosapentaenoic acid (EPA) and DHA give rise to eicosanoids, or cell signaling molecules, which are generally anti-inflammatory in nature, whereas the eicosanoids derived from the omega-6 fatty acids, including arachidonic acid (ARA), are more proinflammatory. DHA and EPA are derived from α-linolenic acid, an essential fatty acid, whereas ARA is derived from linoleic acid, another essential fatty acid. The omega-6 fatty acids are precursors for proinflammatory mediators such as the n-4 series of leukotrienes, whereas the omega-3 fatty acids are precursors for prostaglandins and thromboxanes of the n-3 series and leukotrienes of the n-5 series, which reduce platelet aggregation and vascular tone. The omega-3 fatty acids also generate resolvins, which are endogenous mediators thought to regulate inflammation[16] (**Fig. 1**).

DHA and EPA exert many anti-inflammatory effects, as demonstrated in cell culture models. In human kidney cells, both of these fatty acids decreased gram-negative

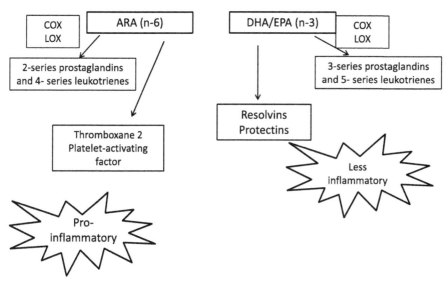

Fig. 1. LCPUFA. Omega-3 and omega-6 LCPUFA compete for cyclo-oxygenase (COX) and lipo-oxygenase (LOX). Depending on the availability of omega-3 LCPUFA, the balance will be shifted toward production of more proinflammatory or less inflammatory eicosanoids.

lipopolysaccharide (LPS)-induced nuclear factor-kappaB (NF-κB) activation,[17] a downstream event inherent to the NEC inflammatory cascade. In a separate study, treatment of human fetal intestinal cells with DHA, EPA, and ARA significantly attenuated proinflammatory cytokine production.[18] Specifically, DHA significantly reduced interleukin-1β (IL-1β)–induced IL-8 and IL-6 protein production compared with controls. Furthermore, DHA treatment of RAW macrophages led to an increase in resolvins, and these resolvins were able to inhibit LPS-induced proinflammatory cytokine expression.[19]

Animal Studies of Necrotizing Enterocolitis

Furthermore, animal models support the role of fish oil in reducing inflammation and modulating the risk for NEC. Using a neonatal rat model of NEC, the authors found a statistically significant reduction in NEC incidence using 3 separate polyunsaturated fatty acids (PUFA)-supplemented formulas, compared with controls ($P<.01$).[20] In a separate study, preterm rats were fed DHA-enriched or EPA-enriched diets compared with a control diet and then subjected to an NEC protocol. Compared with a baseline incidence of NEC of 56% in the control group, the DHA-enriched group demonstrated only a 26.7% NEC incidence, and the EPA-enriched group demonstrated a 20% incidence ($P<.05$).[21] Mouse models have similarly shown a reduction in NEC incidence when chow was supplemented with 10% fish oil for 4 weeks.[22] This study also demonstrated a reduction in intestinal platelet activating factor (PAF) levels in fish oil supplemented mice. PAF is a phospholipid mediator that causes bowel necrosis in NEC models.[23]

LCPUFA likely reduce inflammation via multiple mechanisms. In the authors' study, they found that PUFA supplementation downregulated toll-like receptor (TLR) expression.[20] The TLRs are a family of pattern-recognition receptors that have been well described in the pathogenesis of NEC. Previous work has shown that they are upregulated in animal models of NEC[24] and downregulated in mother-fed pups. The authors also found that PUFA supplementation of formula in their neonatal rat model decreased plasma endotoxin levels, intestinal phospholipase A_2 II expression at 24 hours, and platelet-activating receptor expression at 48 hours.[25]

Human Studies of Necrotizing Enterocolitis

In humans, several studies have evaluated the effect of LCPUFA in term and preterm infants. However, these studies have used different formulations of LCPUFA, in different target populations, and with varying dosages, so it is difficult to make firm conclusions about the utility of LCPUFA as a modality for reducing inflammation. Smithers and colleagues[26] did a meta-analysis in 2008 and found that LCPUFA-supplemented infants did not have a lower risk of NEC; however, the included studies were not limited to the more preterm infants, and those infants are the most at risk for developing NEC. A more recent meta-analysis systematically evaluated the relationship between omega-3 LCPUFA and common neonatal adverse outcomes.[27] Based on a subgroup analysis looking at preterm infants less than 32 weeks, the investigators found a trend toward a reduction in NEC risk in those infants treated with LCPUFA (pooled relative risk 0.50, 95% confidence interval 0.23–1.10). However, of the 18 randomized trials and 6 observational studies included in the meta-analysis, only 5 specifically looked at infants less than 32 weeks, and NEC was not the primary outcome of interest in the included studies.

More specifically, O'Connor and colleagues[28] randomized 470 preterm infants weighing 750 to 1800 g to one of 3 feeding groups. Two groups were supplemented with ARA and DHA and compared with control. These investigators did not report a difference in NEC in any of the treatment groups, but the study was powered to detect a neurodevelopmental outcome rather than NEC. Furthermore, the DHA dose used in this study was 0.27% and 0.24% of fatty acids in the 2 treatment groups, which is a lower dose than used in other studies. A separate study randomized infants less than 35 weeks' gestation to control formula, formula supplemented with algal-DHA and ARA, or formula supplemented with fish oil DHA and algal DHA.[29] There was no difference in comparison of NEC incidence in any of the groups (control 3% vs algal-DHA 5% vs fish oil DHA 5%). Infants less than 37 weeks' gestation were enrolled into a randomized controlled trial in the United Kingdom, and randomized to either a control formula or a formula supplemented with egg lipid LCPUFA.[30] The primary outcome for this study was neurodevelopmental outcome, but the investigators compared rates for common neonatal morbidities. They found no difference in NEC incidence, with 11% of infants in the control formula group and 19% of infants in the experimental formula group reported to have suspected or confirmed NEC. The same group enrolled infants into a separate study using borage oil supplementation, which contains γ-linolenic acid, a precursor of ARA.[31] Eligible infants had a birth weight of less than 2 kg and were less than 35 weeks' gestation. They were randomized to LCPUFA-supplemented formula and compared with control, and the primary outcome was neurodevelopmental outcome at 18 months as measured by the Bayley Scales of Infant Development II. No difference was noted in the secondary outcome of NEC (2% controls vs 4% in experimental formula group). Of note, the infants in this study were eligible even if they received partial mother's own milk, so this may have confounded results.

More recently, several studies in Australia have evaluated various dosing strategies for LCPUFA supplementation. Collins and colleagues[32] randomized a small group of preterm infants born at less than 30 weeks' gestation to several doses of DHA supplementation and compared them with maternal supplementation and placebo. There was no difference noted in NEC incidence. The same group published a separate study in which they randomized preterm infants born before 29 weeks' gestation to 60 mg/kg/d of DHA and compared with placebo, to evaluate the effect on BPD.[33] NEC incidence was the same in both groups. The Docosahexaenoic Acid for the Improvement of Neurodevelopmental Outcome in Preterm Infants (DINO) trial enrolled 657 infants born at less than 33 weeks' gestation and randomized them to supplementation with high-dose DHA (1% total fatty acids) or standard-dose DHA (0.3% total fatty acids).[6] The primary outcome of this study was also to evaluate the effect on neurodevelopmental outcome, but NEC was evaluated as a secondary outcome. Again, there was not a statistical difference, but there was not a comparison group that did not receive DHA.

In a separate study by Carlson and colleagues,[34] infants less than 32 weeks' gestation and 725 to 1375 g at birth whose mothers chose not to breast feed were randomly assigned to one of 2 formulas, either a control formula or one that was supplemented with egg phospholipid, containing 0.13% DHA and 0.41% ARA. Compared with infants fed the control formula, infants who were fed the egg phospholipid–containing formula had a significantly lower incidence of NEC (2.9% experimental formula vs 17.6% control formula, $P<.05$). More recently, a randomized controlled trial in Norway evaluated 141 infants with birth weight less than 1500 g and supplementation with DHA and ARA as compared with control, with the primary outcome of cognitive development, as assessed by the Ages and Stages Questionnaire as well as an assessment of memory.[4] These infants were fed human milk and provided LCPUFA supplementation as study oil. With regards to NEC, no significant difference was noted between groups, and the incidence was low in both groups (1.5% in intervention group vs 3% in control group). Finally, Innis and colleagues[35] evaluated a group of premature infants in a double-blind, randomized, multicenter trial. These investigators randomized infants born weighing less than 1560 g who were to be fed formula to one of 3 formulas. One formula contained DHA alone; one had a combination of DHA and ARA, and the control formula had neither DHA nor ARA. The primary outcome was predetermined to be a comparison of growth and visual acuity, but the investigators also collected information on morbidities such as NEC. As in the aforementioned study, the incidence of NEC was quite low, affecting only one baby out of 62 in the control group, 2 of 66 in the DHA supplemented group, and 0 of 66 in the DHA and ARA supplemented group. No statistical difference was noted.

DISCUSSION

Considering the anti-inflammatory effects of the omega-3 LCPUFA, it is plausible that they may have the potential to modulate inflammation in preterm infants. Modulating inflammation may translate to prevention of inflammatory diseases known to affect preterm infants, such as BPD, sepsis, and NEC.

To date, only one single-center human trial has shown a reduction in NEC incidence after LCPUFA supplementation.[34] However, meta-analysis suggests that LCPUFA may reduce NEC. Additional data are needed, with emphasis on very low-birth-weight infants (VLBW; birth weight <1500 g), the most vulnerable population at risk for NEC.

To date, numerous studies have evaluated LCPUFA supplementation in preterm infants, but the primary outcome has largely been neurodevelopmental. Several studies have evaluated NEC as a secondary outcome, and meta-analyses suggest that LCPUFA may reduce the incidence of NEC. In order to more fully elucidate the potential for LCPUFA to modulate inflammation and affect NEC incidence in at-risk preterm infants, a much larger trial is needed, focusing on only the VLBW infants.

There is biologic plausibility that omega-3 LCPUFA can reduce inflammation and potentially modify NEC risk. Animal studies using established NEC models have shown a reduction in NEC, and the omega-3 LCPUFA exert many anti-inflammatory effects. This effect on inflammation likely occurs via several mechanisms, including production of anti-inflammatory eicosanoids, incorporation of omega-3 LCPUFA into membrane phospholipids, production of anti-inflammatory cytokines, and production of resolvins and protectins (**Fig. 2**).

Both omega-6 and omega-3 LCPUFA produce eicosanoids. However, those produced by omega-3 LCPUFA are much less inflammatory than those produced by omega-6 LCPUFA. Both EPA and ARA use same enzymatic pathways (namely cyclo-oxygenase and lipo-oxygenase) in order to generate prostaglandins, leukotrienes, and thromboxanes.[36] The eicosanoids generated by omega-3 LCPUFA such as EPA, however, are much less inflammatory. Furthermore, supplementation with omega-3 LCPUFA leads to incorporation of these compounds into membrane phospholipids, often replacing ARA, thus limiting its availability for use in production of proinflammatory eicosanoids.

LCPUFA can also modulate inflammation by inhibiting production of proinflammatory cytokines. DHA was shown to reduce IL-1α–induced IL-6 and IL-8 secretion in endothelial cells.[37] Separately, an omega-3 emulsion reduced LPS-induced tumor necrosis factor-α production in RAW macrophages.[38] In this same study, the investigators report a reduction in inhibitor of kappa B (IκB) phosphorylation, and also a reduction in NF-κB activation, both in cells pretreated with the omega-3 emulsion. NF-κB translocates to the nucleus in inflammatory signaling to turn on expression of proinflammatory cytokines, and IκB inhibits this process. In order for NF-κB translocation to occur, IκB must first be phosphorylated. Thus, a reduction in IκB phosphorylation and a reduction in NF-κB activation will effectively blunt proinflammatory cytokine signaling. Furthermore, recent work suggests that peroxisome proliferator–activated receptor alpha (PPARα), a nuclear receptor transcription

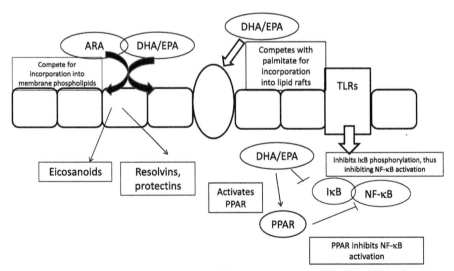

Fig. 2. Potential mechanism of action for fish oil to attenuate inflammation and prevent NEC. Suggested mechanisms include competition for incorporation into membrane phospholipids, competition with palmitate for incorporation into lipid rafts, and inhibition of proinflammatory cytokine production via effects on NF-κB signaling.

factor, is activated by omega-3 LCPUFAs.[39,40] PPARα inhibits NF-κB activation, thus providing another mechanism whereby omega-3 LCPUFAs can reduce inflammation.

LCPUFA can also alter palmitoylation, a posttranslational modification required for effective signaling by many G protein–coupled receptors, including PAF receptor. Palmitoylation targets specific proteins to specialized areas of the plasma membrane called lipid rafts, enabling effective signal transduction. The authors have previously reported that LCPUFA disrupts palmitoylation at least in part, inhibiting PAF receptor signaling.[41]

Last, recent evidence supports the role of resolvins and protectins, mediators derived from omega-3 LCPUFA. These mediators are present especially during the resolution phase of inflammation. They have been shown to reduce inflammatory cytokine expression and reduce neutrophil migration.[19,42]

Despite an abundance of literature supporting the anti-inflammatory role of omega-3 LCPUFA, data for the role of these compounds as prevention for NEC are limited. However, evidence does support their role in prevention of other inflammatory diseases. A recent study by Bisgaard and colleagues[43] supplemented pregnant mothers with fish oil and compared them with placebo-supplemented women. After 3 years, the offspring of the women treated with fish oil had a significantly lower rate of persistent wheezing or asthma (16.9% in fish oil group vs 23.7% in placebo group, $P = .035$). However, this finding has not been supported in similar trials. The DOMInO trial randomized pregnant women to fish oil capsules or vegetable oil capsules without omega-3 LCPUFA.[44] In the follow-up to this trial, the investigators reported on 706 children with a family history of allergic disease. In this particular study, there was no difference in immunoglobulin E–associated allergic disease between the treatment and placebo group (31.5% in both groups, $P = .73$).[45] However, the Bisgaard study used a much higher dose of fish oil (2.4 g), and evidence suggests higher doses are likely necessary in order to exert an anti-inflammatory effect.[46] In further analysis of the DINO trial, the investigators reported on respiratory and allergic outcomes in their study subjects.[47] In those infants treated with high-dose DHA, there was a reduction in BPD both in boys (18.7% high-dose group vs 28% standard-dose group, $P = .03$) and in all infants born at less than 1250 g (34.5% high-dose group vs 47% standard-dose group, $P = .04$). Furthermore, the high-dose group had less hay fever reported at either 12 or 18 months (3.5% high-dose group vs 8.6% standard-dose group, $P = .03$).

Furthermore, low omega-3 LCPUFA levels have been shown to be correlated with common inflammatory morbidities in preterm infants, such as BPD and sepsis.[8,48] In these studies, the omega-6 to omega-3 ratio also correlates with a higher incidence of inflammatory diseases, lending support to the theory that the balance of proinflammatory versus anti-inflammatory mediators contributes to pathogenesis of disease in at-risk infants.

In conclusion, evidence suggests that omega-3 LCPUFA supplementation in preterm infants may lower risk for common inflammatory morbidities in the NICU. However, the human studies to date have used differing products and dosages, making meaningful meta-analyses difficult. Large, multicenter, randomized trials are greatly needed to assess the potential benefit of these compounds. Furthermore, varying doses should be studied, including high doses, because research suggests that the anti-inflammatory benefit may be more robust when giving high-dose LCPUFA. With the survival of smaller and more preterm infants, NEC continues to cause significant morbidity and mortality, and preventative measures are greatly needed.

Best practices

What is the current practice for neonatal necrotizing enterocolitis?

- Preventative measures such as provision of human milk; cautious advancement of feeds
- Recognize signs and symptoms and make prompt diagnosis
- Decompress intestine; withhold enteral feedings; obtain blood culture and start antibiotics; supportive care; surgery as indicated

What changes in current practice are likely to improve outcome?

- Ongoing research into preventative measures to reduce NEC incidence
- Encouragement to mothers to provide mother's own milk as feasible
- Clinical trials into use of LCPUFA, probiotics, growth factors for prevention of NEC

Major recommendations

- Encourage all mothers to provide breast milk for their preterm infants when feasible
- When mother is unable to provide expressed breast milk, encourage use of donor human milk
- Recognize signs and symptoms of NEC promptly and initiate treatment and supportive care
- Continue investigative efforts into preventative measures for reducing NEC incidence

---

REFERENCES

1. Robinson DT, Carlson SE, Murthy K, et al. Docosahexaenoic and arachidonic acid levels in extremely low birth weight infants with prolonged exposure to intravenous lipids. J Pediatr 2013;162(1):56–61.
2. Carlson SE, Werkman SH, Tolley EA. Effect of long-chain n-3 fatty acid supplementation on visual acuity and growth of preterm infants with and without bronchopulmonary dysplasia. Am J Clin Nutr 1996;63(5):687–97.
3. Birch EE, Birch DG, Hoffman DR, et al. Dietary essential fatty acid supply and visual acuity development. Invest Ophthalmol Vis Sci 1992;33(11):3242–53.
4. Henriksen C, Haugholt K, Lindgren M, et al. Improved cognitive development among preterm infants attributable to early supplementation of human milk with docosahexaenoic acid and arachidonic acid. Pediatrics 2008;121(6):1137–45.
5. Birch EE, Garfield S, Hoffman DR, et al. A randomized controlled trial of early dietary supply of long-chain polyunsaturated fatty acids and mental development in term infants. Dev Med Child Neurol 2000;42(3):174–81.
6. Makrides M, Gibson RA, McPhee AJ, et al. Neurodevelopmental outcomes of preterm infants fed high-dose docosahexaenoic acid: a randomized controlled trial. JAMA 2009;301(2):175–82.
7. Carlson SE, Colombo J. Docosahexaenoic acid and arachidonic acid nutrition in early development. Adv Pediatr 2016;63(1):453–71.
8. Martin CR, Dasilva DA, Cluette-Brown JE, et al. Decreased postnatal docosahexaenoic and arachidonic acid blood levels in premature infants are associated with neonatal morbidities. J Pediatr 2011;159(5):743–9.e1-2.
9. Lin HC, Hsu CH, Chen HL, et al. Oral probiotics prevent necrotizing enterocolitis in very low birth weight preterm infants: a multicenter, randomized, controlled trial. Pediatrics 2008;122(4):693–700.
10. Bin-Nun A, Bromiker R, Wilschanski M, et al. Oral probiotics prevent necrotizing enterocolitis in very low birth weight neonates. J Pediatr 2005;147(2):192–6.

11. Costeloe K, Bowler U, Brocklehurst P, et al. A randomised controlled trial of the probiotic Bifidobacterium breve BBG-001 in preterm babies to prevent sepsis, necrotising enterocolitis and death: the Probiotics in Preterm infantS (PiPS) trial. Health Technol Assess 2016;20(66):1–194.

12. Manzoni P, Meyer M, Stolfi I, et al. Bovine lactoferrin supplementation for prevention of necrotizing enterocolitis in very-low-birth-weight neonates: a randomized clinical trial. Early Hum Dev 2014;90(Suppl 1):S60–5.

13. Ledbetter DJ, Juul SE. Erythropoietin and the incidence of necrotizing enterocolitis in infants with very low birth weight. J Pediatr Surg 2000;35(2):178–81 [discussion: 182].

14. Isani M, Illingworth L, Herman E, et al. Soybean-derived recombinant human epidermal growth factor protects against experimental necrotizing enterocolitis. J Pediatr Surg 2018;53(6):1203–7.

15. Feng J, El-Assal ON, Besner GE. Heparin-binding epidermal growth factor-like growth factor decreases the incidence of necrotizing enterocolitis in neonatal rats. J Pediatr Surg 2006;41(1):144–9 [discussion: 144–9].

16. Hong S, Gronert K, Devchand PR, et al. Novel docosatrienes and 17S-resolvins generated from docosahexaenoic acid in murine brain, human blood, and glial cells. Autacoids in anti-inflammation. J Biol Chem 2003;278(17):14677–87.

17. Li H, Ruan XZ, Powis SH, et al. EPA and DHA reduce LPS-induced inflammation responses in HK-2 cells: evidence for a PPAR-gamma-dependent mechanism. Kidney Int 2005;67(3):867–74.

18. Wijendran V, Brenna JT, Wang DH, et al. Long-chain polyunsaturated fatty acids attenuate the IL-1beta-induced proinflammatory response in human fetal intestinal epithelial cells. Pediatr Res 2015;78(6):626–33.

19. Caron JP, Gandy JC, Brown JL, et al. Docosahexaenoic acid-derived oxidized lipid metabolites modulate the inflammatory response of lipolysaccharide-stimulated macrophages. Prostaglandins Other Lipid Mediat 2018;136:76–83.

20. Lu J, Jilling T, Li D, et al. Polyunsaturated fatty acid supplementation alters proinflammatory gene expression and reduces the incidence of necrotizing enterocolitis in a neonatal rat model. Pediatr Res 2007;61(4):427–32.

21. Ohtsuka Y, Okada K, Yamakawa Y, et al. omega-3 fatty acids attenuate mucosal inflammation in premature rat pups. J Pediatr Surg 2011;46(3):489–95.

22. Akisu M, Baka M, Coker I, et al. Effect of dietary n-3 fatty acids on hypoxia-induced necrotizing enterocolitis in young mice. n-3 fatty acids alter platelet-activating factor and leukotriene B4 production in the intestine. Biol Neonate 1998;74(1):31–8.

23. Gonzalez-Crussi F, Hsueh W. Experimental model of ischemic bowel necrosis. The role of platelet-activating factor and endotoxin. Am J Pathol 1983;112(1):127–35.

24. Jilling T, Simon D, Lu J, et al. The roles of bacteria and TLR4 in rat and murine models of necrotizing enterocolitis. J Immunol 2006;177(5):3273–82.

25. Caplan MS, Russell T, Xiao Y, et al. Effect of polyunsaturated fatty acid (PUFA) supplementation on intestinal inflammation and necrotizing enterocolitis (NEC) in a neonatal rat model. Pediatr Res 2001;49(5):647–52.

26. Smithers LG, Gibson RA, McPhee A, et al. Effect of long-chain polyunsaturated fatty acid supplementation of preterm infants on disease risk and neurodevelopment: a systematic review of randomized controlled trials. Am J Clin Nutr 2008;87(4):912–20.

27. Zhang P, Lavoie PM, Lacaze-Masmonteil T, et al. Omega-3 long-chain polyunsaturated fatty acids for extremely preterm infants: a systematic review. Pediatrics 2014;134(1):120–34.

28. O'Connor DL, Hall R, Adamkin D, et al. Growth and development in preterm infants fed long-chain polyunsaturated fatty acids: a prospective, randomized controlled trial. Pediatrics 2001;108(2):359–71.

29. Clandinin MT, Van Aerde JE, Merkel KL, et al. Growth and development of preterm infants fed infant formulas containing docosahexaenoic acid and arachidonic acid. J Pediatr 2005;146(4):461–8.

30. Fewtrell MS, Morley R, Abbott RA, et al. Double-blind, randomized trial of long-chain polyunsaturated fatty acid supplementation in formula fed to preterm infants. Pediatrics 2002;110(1 Pt 1):73–82.

31. Fewtrell MS, Abbott RA, Kennedy K, et al. Randomized, double-blind trial of long-chain polyunsaturated fatty acid supplementation with fish oil and borage oil in preterm infants. J Pediatr 2004;144(4):471–9.

32. Collins CT, Sullivan TR, McPhee AJ, et al. A dose response randomised controlled trial of docosahexaenoic acid (DHA) in preterm infants. Prostaglandins Leukot Essent Fatty Acids 2015;99:1–6.

33. Collins CT, Makrides M, McPhee AJ, et al. Docosahexaenoic acid and bronchopulmonary dysplasia in preterm infants. N Engl J Med 2017;376(13):1245–55.

34. Carlson SE, Montalto MB, Ponder DL, et al. Lower incidence of necrotizing enterocolitis in infants fed a preterm formula with egg phospholipids. Pediatr Res 1998;44(4):491–8.

35. Innis SM, Adamkin DH, Hall RT, et al. Docosahexaenoic acid and arachidonic acid enhance growth with no adverse effects in preterm infants fed formula. J Pediatr 2002;140(5):547–54.

36. James MJ, Cleland LG, Gibson RA, et al. Interaction between fish and vegetable oils in relation to rat leucocyte leukotriene production. J Nutr 1991;121(5):631–7.

37. De Caterina R, Cybulsky MI, Clinton SK, et al. The omega-3 fatty acid docosahexaenoate reduces cytokine-induced expression of proatherogenic and proinflammatory proteins in human endothelial cells. Arterioscler Thromb 1994;14(11):1829–36.

38. Novak TE, Babcock TA, Jho DH, et al. NF-kappa B inhibition by omega -3 fatty acids modulates LPS-stimulated macrophage TNF-alpha transcription. Am J Physiol Lung Cell Mol Physiol 2003;284(1):L84–9.

39. Tillman EM, Guan P, Howze TJ, et al. Role of PPARalpha in the attenuation of bile acid-induced apoptosis by omega-3 long-chain polyunsaturated fatty acids in cultured hepatocytes. Pediatr Res 2016;79(5):754–8.

40. Chang YF, Hou YC, Pai MH, et al. Effects of omega-3 polyunsaturated fatty acids on the homeostasis of CD4+ T cells and lung injury in mice with polymicrobial sepsis. JPEN J Parenter Enteral Nutr 2017;41(5):805–14.

41. Lu J, Caplan MS, Li D, et al. Polyunsaturated fatty acids block platelet-activating factor-induced phosphatidylinositol 3 kinase/Akt-mediated apoptosis in intestinal epithelial cells. Am J Physiol Gastrointest Liver Physiol 2008;294(5):G1181–90.

42. Bannenberg GL, Chiang N, Ariel A, et al. Molecular circuits of resolution: formation and actions of resolvins and protectins. J Immunol 2005;174(7):4345–55.

43. Bisgaard H, Stokholm J, Chawes BL, et al. Fish oil-derived fatty acids in pregnancy and wheeze and asthma in offspring. N Engl J Med 2016;375(26):2530–9.

44. Makrides M, Gibson RA, McPhee AJ, et al. Effect of DHA supplementation during pregnancy on maternal depression and neurodevelopment of young children: a randomized controlled trial. JAMA 2010;304(15):1675–83.

45. Best KP, Sullivan T, Palmer D, et al. Prenatal fish oil supplementation and allergy: 6-year follow-up of a randomized controlled trial. Pediatrics 2016;137(6) [pii: e20154443].
46. Lapillonne A, Moltu SJ. Long-chain polyunsaturated fatty acids and clinical outcomes of preterm infants. Ann Nutr Metab 2016;69(Suppl 1):35–44.
47. Manley BJ, Makrides M, Collins CT, et al. High-dose docosahexaenoic acid supplementation of preterm infants: respiratory and allergy outcomes. Pediatrics 2011;128(1):e71–7.
48. Fares S, Sethom MM, Kacem S, et al. Plasma arachidonic and docosahexaenoic acids in Tunisian very low birth weight infants: status and association with selected neonatal morbidities. J Health Popul Nutr 2015;33:1.

Oropharyngeal Mother's Milk

State of the Science and Influence on Necrotizing Enterocolitis

Nancy A. Garofalo, PhD, APRN, NNP[a,b],*, Michael S. Caplan, MD[a,b]

KEYWORDS

- Mother's own milk • Breastmilk • Human milk • Oropharyngeal • Oral immune
- Oral care • Premature • NEC • Oropharyngeal milk • Oropharyngeal colostrum
- Oropharyngeal therapy

KEY POINTS

- Extremely low birth weight infants experience a lack of oropharyngeal exposure to protective biofactors after birth, a deficit that may be contributing to necrotizing enterocolitis pathogenesis.
- Oropharyngeal mother's milk can serve as an immunomodulatory therapy, an adjunct to enteral feeds of mother's milk administered via a nasogastric or orogastric tube.
- Oropharyngeal therapy with mother's own milk may serve to (ex utero) mimic the protective effects of amniotic fluid for the extremely low birth weight infant, providing protection against necrotizing enterocolitis.

INTRODUCTION

Amniotic fluid and mother's own milk (MOM) are 2 immunoprotective body fluids that are intended to be in close contact with the fetus and newborn's oropharynx. In utero, amniotic fluid exposes the fetus to protective biofactors, which stimulate the immune system and promote intestinal maturation. After birth, MOM provides a continuum of beneficial effects providing oropharyngeal biofactor exposure and facilitating transition to extrauterine life. In a term pregnancy, the fetus receives uninterrupted biofactor exposure until 40 completed weeks of gestation. After birth, the term breastfed newborn receives continued oropharyngeal biofactor exposure with every feeding. Whereas a healthy term newborn receives this natural protection, an extremely low birth weight (ELBW) infant does not.

Disclosure Statement: N.A. Garofalo has nothing to disclose.
[a] Department of Pediatrics, NorthShore University HealthSystem, Evanston Hospital, 2650 Ridge Avenue, Evanston, IL 60201, USA; [b] Pritzker School of Medicine, University of Chicago, Chicago, IL, USA
* Corresponding author.
E-mail address: ngarofalo@northshore.org

With a preterm delivery, amniotic fluid exposure stops abruptly, and the ELBW infant's oropharynx is no longer exposed to protective biofactors. Whereas MOM contains many protective biofactors, the infant's oropharynx remains unexposed to this natural protection (for up ≤10 weeks), because milk feedings are given via a nasogastric tube, which bypasses the infant's oropharynx. The absence of oropharyngeal exposure to protective biofactors during this critical period after birth may be contributing substantially to NEC risk and pathogenesis. Oropharyngeal administration of mother's milk may serve to mimic the protective effects of amniotic fluid, potentially protecting against NEC. This article presents evidence to support the biological plausibility for the use of oropharyngeal mother's milk as an adjunctive immunomodulatory therapy to protect premature infants against NEC.

BODY
Extremely Low Birth Weight Infants and the Risk for Necrotizing Enterocolitis

ELBW (birthweight of <1000 g) infants represent a small (only 1% of annual US births)[1] population, however they account for 23% of total neonatal health care costs annually.[2] Mortality is substantial and survivors suffer from prematurity-associated infectious morbidities,[3] including NEC, which is a potentially lethal gastrointestinal infectious and inflammatory disorder. NEC is associated with long-term morbidities, including severe neurologic impairment,[4] which create a massive financial burden for families and society. NEC accounts for an estimated $1 billion in health care dollars yearly.[5] The risk of NEC is inversely related to birthweight; therefore, ELBW infants have the highest incidence (≤15%), the most severe course of the disease, and the highest NEC-associated mortality rates (30%).[4,5] The development of preventative strategies, beginning with the first days of life, is an urgent clinical priority.

NEC pathophysiology includes altered intestinal microbiota (dysbiosis), mucosal injury, impaired host defense, an unbalanced proinflammatory response, and cellular necrosis.[6] A central component in the pathogenesis of NEC seems to be a pathogen-predominant microbiota, which allows for bacterial translocation and injury to the fragile and immature mucosal barrier. Compared with a healthy term infant, the ELBW infant has reduced bacterial diversity, decreased commensal organisms, and a predominance of pathogens.[7] The long-term exposure to hospital pathogens, delayed initiation of enteral feeds, exposure to antibiotics, and the presence of endotracheal tubes, umbilical and central lines, suction catheters, and nasogastric tubes are factors that decrease microbial diversity and promote dysbiosis for the ELBW infant.[8] Immaturity in intrinsic intestinal host mechanisms including B and T lymphocytes, levels of secretory IgA (sIgA), intestinal motility, gastric acid, proteolytic enzymes, intestinal mucus, surface glycoconjugates, and epithelial membrane tight junctions promote mucosal injury, which facilitates the proliferation and translocation of pathogens, and their endotoxins, into the blood stream. The response of the immature enterocyte to pathogens results in exaggerated proinflammatory signaling and together with impaired antiinflammatory activity leads to tissue injury, release of oxygen free radicals leading to further cellular injury, and perpetuation of the inflammatory cascade. An unbalanced proinflammatory response and an abnormal host defense leads to the rapid progression of this lethal disease, with areas of ulceration and necrotic tissue potentially leading to perforation of the bowel and subsequent peritonitis.[6-8] In severe cases, NEC leads to multisystem organ failure and death.

Protection Against Necrotizing Enterocolitis with Mother's Milk Feedings

Feedings of MOM have been linked with a lower incidence and severity of NEC in premature infants.[9-14] Even a daily dose of at least 50 mL/kg/d of mother's milk feedings, during a critical period after birth, can significantly reduce the risk of NEC for premature infants.[12–14]

The protection against NEC with mother's milk feedings is attributed to a plethora of milk biofactors, which include hormones, enzymes, soluble CD14, immunoglobulins including sIgA, antiinflammatory cytokines including interleukin-10 (IL-10), platelet-activating factor acetylhydrolase, antioxidants (including vitamin E, carotene, and glutathione), glycoproteins including lactoferrin, lysozyme, human milk oligosaccharides, polyunsaturated fatty acids, erythropoietin, glutamine, nucleotides, and (intestinal) growth factors including transforming growth factor-beta (TGF-β), epidermal growth factor (EGF), and heparin-binding EGF-like growth factor.[15–18] Collectively, milk biofactors can protect against NEC by increasing commensal bacteria, preventing the colonization and proliferation of pathogens, preventing bacterial translocation, balancing the inflammatory response, providing antioxidant protection, decreasing epithelial permeability, maintaining the integrity of the intestinal epithelial barrier and healing areas of injured mucosa, promoting intestinal growth, maturation and motility, and regulating the immune response.[15–18] Many of these protective components are decreased with freezing, thawing and storage practices that are routinely used in the NICU, and it has been suggested that fresh human milk may be more protective than processed aliquots.

Amniotic Fluid and Preterm Colostrum: Implications for the Extremely Low Birth Weight Infant

In utero, the fetus swallows up to 200 mL/kg/d of bacteriostatic amniotic fluid. This intake provides the fetus with direct oropharyngeal exposure to many protective (immune and trophic) biofactors, contained in amniotic fluid, including immunoglobulins (ie, sIgA), cytokines, glycoproteins (ie, lactoferrin) and intestinal trophic factors (ie, EGF and TGF-β), among others. During the final trimester of pregnancy, the weight of the intestinal mucosa increases by more than 50%,[19] and this rapid growth is attributed to the abundance of growth factors in the amniotic fluid during this period of gestation.

ELBW infants are born before the last trimester of pregnancy and experience a sudden termination of amniotic fluid exposure. The infant's oropharynx is no longer exposed to protective biofactors, which stimulate the immune system and promote intestinal maturation. Many biofactors are also contained in MOM, with the highest concentrations found in the milk expressed by mothers of ELBW infants—preterm milk. Although the highest concentrations are found in early milk (colostrum), the levels of many protective biofactors remain high in preterm milk for several weeks after delivery.[20–22] These gestation-specific trends in biofactor concentrations suggest that preterm milk is uniquely suited to facilitate extrauterine transition, and protect the ELBW infant against infection, during the first weeks of life. However, because of clinical instability, ELBW infants are either not fed enterally for several days after birth or are fed only minimal amounts. This critical "exposure" period is a time during which the (adequate exposure) provision of MOM may significantly improve health outcomes. Postbirth fasting leads to intestinal atrophy and dysbiosis, which contribute to the pathogenesis of NEC.

Per oral feeds are not introduced until at least 32 weeks corrected gestational age, and enteral feeds are administered via a nasogastric or orogastric tube, which bypasses the infant's oropharynx. Thus, oropharyngeal exposure to protective (milk) biofactors is delayed for up to 10 weeks for the least mature ELBW infants. Unfortunately, it is not uncommon for mothers of ELBW infants to discontinue milk expression during this prolonged period of time because they become discouraged with their low milk volume. When formula is given for per oral feeds at 32 weeks corrected gestational age, because mother's milk is no longer available, the ELBW infant's oropharynx is never exposed to protective biofactors after birth. This deficit has never been addressed in neonatal practice. In a normal term pregnancy, the fetus received uninterrupted (biofactor) exposure until 40 completed weeks of gestation. It is plausible that this deficit—the lack of oropharyngeal exposure to protective biofactors after birth—may be contributing substantially to prematurity-associated infectious morbidities for the ELBW infant, particularly NEC. Oropharyngeal mother's milk is a natural substitute for amniotic fluid exposure and stimulates immune responses that are separate and distinct from enteral exposure.

Mechanisms for Protection Against Necrotizing Enterocolitis with Oropharyngeal Mother's Milk

Oropharyngeal mother's milk may be protective against NEC via several mechanisms: (1) interaction of milk cytokines with oropharyngeal-associated lymphoid tissue immune cells, (2) mucosal absorption of protective biofactors, (3) barrier protection against pathogens, (4) local and systemic effects of oligosaccharides, (5) antiinflammatory protection, and (6) protective effects of antioxidants. These mechanisms are explained herein and depicted in **Fig. 1**.

Interaction of milk cytokines with oropharyngeal-associated lymphoid tissue immune cells

Studies with small and large animals, and human subjects, have shown that the oropharyngeal route can be used to administer cytokines safely and effectively. The cytokines can have a stimulatory effect on the oropharyngeal-associated lymphoid tissue system, resulting in T-cell activation and systemic dissemination leading to a variety of end-organ immune responses.[15,16] An oropharyngeal-associated lymphoid tissue-associated stimulus can result in immune activation at distant organs, or an antiinflammatory response, based on the cytokines released and the types of immune cells along the signaling pathway. When cytokines (IL-2, -12, -15, and -18) are administered onto the oral mucosa of mice, they interact with immune cells in the oropharyngeal lymphoid or epithelial tissue, with subsequent cell-to-cell signaling that results in

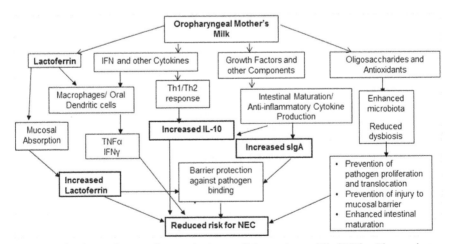

Fig. 1. Mechanisms of protection against necrotizing enterocolitis (NEC) with oropharyngeal mother's milk. IFNγ, interferon-γ; sIgA, secretory immunoglobulin A; Th1/Th2, T-helper 1/T-helper 2; TNFα, tumor necrosis factor alpha.

a systemic response.[23] Milk cytokines may exert a similar cell-to-cell effect by interacting with the epithelial, dendritic, or lymphoid cells in the infant's oropharyngeal-associated lymphoid tissue providing systemic, protective immunostimulatory effects. Other milk biofactors, including sIgA, lysozyme, and macrophages, may also be involved in oropharyngeal-associated lymphoid tissue cellular signaling because these developmental messages are thought to occur through leukocytes, hormones, growth factors, lactoferrin, and oligosaccharides.[24]

Mucosal absorption of protective biofactors

Many milk biofactors can be systemically absorbed, including growth factors, glycoproteins (such as lactoferrin), immunoglobulins (such as sIgA), oligosaccharides, cytokines, and fatty acids. These macromolecules can be absorbed intact into the circulation, which suggests protection against systemic infection. With oropharyngeal mother's milk, intestinal growth factors (eg, EGF, TGF-β) may be absorbed mucosally or may travel to the gastrointestinal tract and provide local maturational effects. Several growth factors are significantly more concentrated in mother's milk, as compared with amniotic fluid. For example, TGF-β levels are lowest in amniotic fluid (5.0 ng/mL) compared with mature milk (950 ng/mL), but highest in colostrum (1366 ng/mL).[25] Therefore, even small drops of milk can provide a "dose" equivalent to amniotic fluid exposure.

Oligosaccharides may be also absorbed mucosally with systemic effects that are protective against NEC; including immunomodulatory functions, stimulating immune maturation, and antiinflammatory effects.[26] With oropharyngeal mother's milk, some oligosaccharides may also travel to the gut where they can help to maintain intestinal integrity, promote intestinal development, and enhance the microbiome through prebiotic effects on *Bifidobacteria* spp. growth, as described elsewhere in this article.

Lactoferrin is an iron-binding glycoprotein that can also be absorbed mucosally, and has numerous protective functions including antimicrobial, antiinflammatory, immunomodulatory, and antioxidant properties.[27] With oropharyngeal mother's milk, some lactoferrin may travel to the gut, where it provides antiinflammatory effects and can protect the intestinal mucosa from injury. Lactoferrin can also protect against NEC by attenuating oxidative damage to intestinal epithelial cells.

Barrier protection against pathogens

Components in mother's milk that provide barrier protection include oligosaccharides, lactoferrin, and sIgA. Oligosaccharides serve as decoy receptors to competitively bind and inhibit pathogens. Lactoferrin and sIgA promote mucosal immunity. They prevent the attachment of pathogens, and/or their toxins, to epithelial cell surface receptors. By inhibiting pathogen binding, they protect the mucosal barrier from injury, maintain intestinal integrity, and prevent bacterial translocation, protecting against NEC. Lactoferrin also has antiinflammatory and mucosal healing properties that serve to protect against NEC.

Local and systemic effects of oligosaccharides

Oligosaccharides have prebiotic effects and stimulate the growth of nonpathogenic Bifidobacteria. By promoting commensal bacteria colonization, oligosaccharides prevent pathogen colonization, proliferation, and translocation. They maintain intestinal integrity and promote intestinal maturation through direct interactions with epithelial cells.

Antiinflammatory protection

Antiinflammatory biofactors contained in mother's milk include cytokines, soluble cytokine receptors, K-casein, lactoferrin, polyunsaturated fatty acids, nucleotides, hormones, and growth factors. Platelet-activating factor acetylhydrolase provides antiinflammatory protection against NEC, by degrading platelet activating factor, a proinflammatory mediator in NEC pathogenesis. IL-10 is a potent antiinflammatory cytokine that helps to maintain the integrity of the mucosal barrier and heals areas of injury, protecting against NEC. Oligosaccharides, polyunsaturated fatty acids, growth factors, and specific cytokines contained in mother's milk promote IL-10 production. Nucleotides also provide antiinflammatory protection against NEC. Antiinflammatory milk components modulate the infant's immune response and may also travel to the gut, where they can protect the intestine from inflammation and mucosal injury, decreasing the risk for NEC.

Protective effects of antioxidants

The immature intestinal mucosa is vulnerable to injury from oxidative stress, which contributes to NEC pathogenesis. Milk antioxidants (ie, peroxidase, catalase, superoxide dismutate, glutathione, vitamins E and C, beta-carotene, lactoferrin) protect against free radical damage by reactive oxygen species. ELBW infants have an immature antioxidant defense system, and require supplemental oxygen, which increases their risk for oxidative stress-derived diseases. With oropharyngeal mother's milk, antioxidants may directly protect immune cells in the oropharynx and also may travel to the gut protecting the mucosal barrier from oxidative injury, preventing oxidative stress-induced changes in the gut microbiota, reducing inflammation, and preventing pathogen translocation, all of which protect against NEC.[15]

Evidence to Support the Use of Oropharyngeal Mother's Milk as an Immune Therapy

Oropharyngeal mother's milk for ELBW infants was first introduced into the medical literature in 2009,[28] and 2 small feasibility pilot studies soon followed.[29,30] A small randomized controlled trial (n = 16)[31] showed beneficial immune effects for ELBW infants who received 0.2 mL of own mother's colostrum administered oropharyngeally every 2 hours for 48 consecutive hours compared with placebo-treated controls. For infants in the treatment group, a large effect size (1.30) was noted for urinary lactoferrin, which suggests that results may have reached statistical significance with a larger sample. Milk-treated infants reached full enteral feedings (150 mL/kg/d) on average 10 days earlier (14.3 $\pm$ 5.7 days vs 24.2 $\pm$ 8.7 days; P = .032) compared with placebo-treated controls.[31] Findings from recent studies suggest many potential benefits for premature infants who receive this intervention, including enhanced immune status (higher concentrations of serum IgA,[32] urinary sIgA,[33] salivary sIgA,[34] urinary lactoferrin,[35] and salivary lactoferrin[35]), reduced inflammatory markers (lower concentrations of urinary IL-1β, salivary TGF-β-1, and salivary IL-8),[33] a lower risk for clinical sepsis,[33] enhanced oral microbiota,[36,37] a reduced time to achieve full enteral feedings,[35,37,38] and full per oral feedings,[36] improved growth,[38] enhanced breastfeeding outcomes,[39] and a decreased length of hospitalization.[36] Others have incorporated this practice into ventilator-associated pneumonia prevention bundles or feeding protocols; therefore, the effect of the intervention itself cannot be determined.

Techniques, Methods, and Controversies: Implications for Clinical Practice

Based on current evidence, oropharyngeal mother's milk seems to be beneficial to recipient infants and without adverse effects. Yet, despite promising results from recent studies, safety and efficacy have not yet been established in an adequately powered placebo-controlled, randomized trial.

Recent studies are primarily retrospective in design, incorporated small samples, and were not adequately powered to look at clinical outcomes such as NEC. Another limitation is the wide variation in the methodologies for the frequency of treatments (ranging from every 2–6 hours, or on an as-needed basis), the duration of the treatment protocol (ranging from 2 to 7 days), the volume of milk (dose) administered per treatment (ranging from 0.1 to 1.0 mL), the type of applicator (syringe vs swab), and the use of fresh versus frozen milk.[30,32–39]

The terminology used to describe oropharyngeal administration of mother's milk is also quite variable (**Box 1**) in published reports.[30,32–39] However, the underlying concept is the same: placing drops of mother's milk onto the infant's oral mucosa so that (milk) biofactors may provide immunomodulation. Although the initial pilot studies focused on the use of only colostrum (not mature milk) for a very brief (48-hour) treatment period intended for ELBW infants who were nil per os owing to clinical instability, current studies incorporate longer treatment protocols. The latest terminology—oropharyngeal therapy with MOM (OPT-MOM)[40]—describes the use of mother's milk as a natural substitute for biofactor-rich amniotic fluid (oropharyngeal) exposure. OPT-MOM incorporates own mother's milk (colostrum, transitional, and mature milk) administered oropharyngeally, as an immunomodulatory adjunct therapy to nasogastric tube feedings. Beginning as soon as colostrum is available, the infant receives 0.2 mL of own mother's milk administered oropharyngeally every 2 hours for 48 consecutive hours, followed by 0.2 mL every 3 hours until the infant reaches 32 weeks corrected gestational age. The OPT-MOM approach is currently being evaluated in a multicenter randomized controlled trial (funded by the Gerber Foundation)[40] to determine its impact on clinical outcomes, including the incidence of NEC, for extremely premature infants. The OPT-MOM approach is intended to provide sustained immune effects; therefore, the protocol is continued for many weeks after birth until per oral feedings are introduced. A brief 2- to 7-day treatment protocol, as

---

Box 1
Oropharyngeal administration of mother's milk

- Oropharyngeal mother's milk
- Oropharyngeal therapy with mother's own milk
- Administración de calostro orofaríngeo
- Oral colostrum priming
- Oral immune therapy with colostrum
- Oropharyngeal colostrum
- Buccal administration of colostrum
- Colostrum oral care
- Mouth feeds with colostrum
- Buccal swabbing with colostrum
- Colostrum swabbing
- Oral colostrum
- Oral human milk swabbing
- Oral swabbing with colostrum
- Oral care/mouth care with colostrum

described in recent studies, is not likely to impact important clinical outcomes such as NEC. Importantly, these immune benefits may not persist once treatments are stopped, unless the infant is ready to begin per oral feeds of mother's milk.

In a recent study,[37] the investigators suggest that a brief 48-hour treatment protocol may have limited effects on the oral microbiota or clinical outcomes such as ventilator-associated pneumonia, NEC, late-onset sepsis, and chronic lung disease. In a second study,[34] after a treatment protocol that lasted 5 days, the immune benefits that were noted on day of life 7 for milk-treated infants were not sustained when measured 1 week later (day of life 14). The authors concluded that the lack of effect on clinical outcomes may have been due to the short (5-day) duration of the treatment protocol and that the immune effects (higher levels of salivary sIgA) may have been sustained with a longer treatment protocol.[34] In a third recent study,[35] even after a 7-day treatment protocol, immune effects were not sustained. In milk-treated very low birth weight infants, salivary IgA was significantly increased from baseline levels after 7 consecutive days of treatments (0.2 mL every 4 hours), compared with placebo controls ($P = .04$), but these significant differences were not sustained when measured 14 days after the treatment protocol was stopped.[35] Therefore, results from these recent studies suggest that frequent and prolonged dosing, until per oral feeds of mother's milk can be safely introduced, is more likely to provide sustained immune effects and impact health outcomes for recipient infants.

The OPT-MOM approach is intended as an immune therapy; therefore, the milk should be treated as a medication and a precise dose should be administered, using a sterile syringe. With a precise dose (0.2 mL; approximately 8 drops), the infant can consistently receive with each treatment, biofactor doses comparable with in utero exposure. As an example, based on levels of EGF and lactoferrin in human amniotic fluid and also in preterm human milk,[22,41] a fetus weighing 1 kg would be exposed to approximately 38 ng of EGF and 172 µg of lactoferrin daily via amniotic fluid (200 mL/kg fetal weight/d). Using OPT-MOM as a substitute for amniotic fluid exposure, the ELBW infant weighing 1 kg would receive a dose of 396 ng of EGF and 658 µg of lactoferrin with dosing every 2 hours (2.4 mL/d), and 216 ng of EGF and 450 µg of lactoferrin with dosing every 3 hours (1.6 mL/d). In this manner, the OPT-MOM approach can provide the ELBW infant with higher doses of protective biofactors. This finding is important because the ELBW infant remains hospitalized (for ≤4 months) in the pathogen-laden NICU, compared with the sterile in utero environment for the fetus. Because very small volumes (<2.4 mL/d) of milk are needed for OPT-MOM, even mothers with a very low milk volume can easily provide the small amounts needed.

Donor milk is not optimal for oropharyngeal administration. The pasteurization process destroys immune biofactors or significantly decreases their antimicrobial functions; lactoferrin is reduced by 88%.[42] Although enteral feedings of donor milk are beneficial for ELBW infants, own mother's milk should be prioritized for oropharyngeal administration. If only small volumes of colostrum are available in the first days of life, the colostrum should be used for oropharyngeal administration, and donor milk should be used for the initiation of small enteral feeds. To provide the ELBW infant with the same benefits that a breastfed infant would receive, the oropharyngeal milk should be administered in the order that it was expressed, with a gradual progression from colostrum, then transitional, to mature milk.

With any clinical intervention, patient safety and infection control must be a priority. Some hospitals are administering fortified breastmilk via the oropharyngeal route to ELBW infants in the first weeks after birth. The bedside nurse collects the dose of milk at the point of care when the infant's enteral feeding is due. Using a syringe or swab, the bedside nurse collects a small volume of milk from the fortified milk that is stored in the NICU refrigerator and intended for the infant's enteral feeds. This procedure is repeated between 8 and 12 times per day, depending on the infant's feeding regime. This practice raises several concerns. Repeatedly dipping syringes or swabs into the refrigerated milk can easily contaminate the milk with NICU pathogens, placing the infant at risk for infection. In a recent review,[43] up to 40% of milk samples in the NICU were contaminated with pathogenic organisms and the most common were coagulase-negative *Staphylococci*, *Staphylococcus aureus*, and *Enterobacteriaceae*.[43–45] Preventing the contamination of mother's milk must be a clinical priority.

There is no evidence to support the safety of administering oropharyngeal fortified milk to ELBW infants before they reach 32 weeks CGA. In addition to the aforementioned risk for milk contamination with 'point of care' collection of the milk sample, the use of iron-enriched fortifier in the milk may limit the immune benefits of the intervention. For example, (milk) lactoferrin's antimicrobial functions depend on its ability to compete with bacteria for iron-binding sites. In the presence of iron-enriched fortifier, lactoferrin's bioactivity is impaired because iron-saturated lactoferrin has significantly reduced antimicrobial activity.[46,47] In order to maximize the immune benefits of this intervention, only unfortified milk should be utilized.

The OPT-MOM approach is primarily intended for the ELBW population until per oral feeds can be safely introduced. Yet, this intervention is also beneficial for any infant who is unable to feed per oral owing to clinical instability, congenital anomalies including cardiac disease and omphalocele, or postoperative status.[48–50]

SUMMARY

ELBW infants do not receive oropharyngeal exposure to protective milk biofactors until 32 weeks of corrected gestational age, up to 10 weeks after birth for the least mature ELBW infants. This deficit may be contributing to NEC risk and pathogenesis. Oropharyngeal mother's milk, specifically the OPT-MOM approach, may be used to mimic the protective effects of biofactor-rich amniotic fluid exposure after birth for the ELBW infant. For OPT-MOM to serve as a potential adjunctive immune therapy, the dosing must precise, frequent, and sustained until per oral feeds are started. Evidence to date supports biological plausibility for protection against infectious morbidities, especially NEC, using this approach.

Best practices

What is current practice?

- ELBW infants do not receive oropharyngeal exposure to protective milk biofactors for up to 10 weeks after birth.

- MOM is typically administered as a feeding via a nasogastric or orogastric tube, which bypasses the infant's oropharynx.

- Oropharyngeal exposure to protective biofactors cannot occur until per oral feedings of mother's milk are started at 32 weeks corrected gestational age or older.

What changes in practice are likely to improve outcomes?

- Early postbirth oropharyngeal exposure to MOM is likely to improve outcomes for the ELBW infant.

- The uninterrupted continuation of OPT-MOM treatments, until the infant reaches 32 weeks corrected gestational age, is likely to provide sustained immune benefits and reduce NEC risk.

Major recommendations

- Begin OPT-MOM as soon as possible after birth.

- If only a small amount of MOM is available, it should be prioritized for OPT-MOM, and donor milk can be administered via gavage as a feeding.

- To mimic the beneficial effects of amniotic fluid, OPT-MOM dosing must be precise, and treatments must be frequent and sustained until per oral feeds are started.

Summary Statement

The OPT-MOM approach may protect the ELBW infant against NEC, by providing oropharyngeal exposure to protective biofactors, similar to the protective effects a fetus naturally receives via amniotic fluid exposure during the last trimester of pregnancy.

ACKNOWLEDGMENTS

This study was generously supported by the Gerber Foundation (grant ID # 3877).

REFERENCES

1. Hamilton BE, Martin JA, Osterman MJ, et al. Division of vital statistics. Births: final data for 2015. Natl Vital Stat Rep 2016;65:1–15.
2. Gilbert WM, Nesbitt TS, Danielsen B. The cost of prematurity: quantification by gestational age and birth weight. Obstet Gynecol 2003;102:488–92.
3. Stoll BJ, Hansen NI, Bell EF, et al. Neonatal outcomes of extremely preterm infants from the NICHD Neonatal Research Network. Pediatrics 2010;126:443–56.
4. Wadhawan R, Oh W, Hintz SR, et al, NICHD Neonatal Research Network. Neuro-developmental outcomes of extremely low birth weight infants with spontaneous intestinal perforation or surgical necrotizing enterocolitis. J Perinatol 2014;34(1): 64–70.
5. Neu J, Walker WA. Necrotizing enterocolitis. N Engl J Med 2011;364:255–64.
6. Frost BF, Modi R, Caplan MS. New medical and surgical insights into neonatal necrotizing enterocolitis. JAMA Pediatr 2017;171:83–8.
7. Claud EC. Probiotics and neonatal necrotizing enterocolitis. Anaerobe 2011;17: 180–5.
8. Claud EC, Walker WA. Bacterial colonization, probiotics and necrotizing entero-colitis. J Clin Gastroenterol 2008;42:S46–51.
9. Johnson TJ, Patel AL, Bigger HR, et al. Cost savings of human milk as a strategy to reduce the incidence of necrotizing enterocolitis in very low birth weight in-fants. Neonatology 2015;107:271–6.
10. Meinzen-Derr J, Poindexter B, Wrage L, et al. Role of human milk in extremely low birth weight infants' risk of necrotizing enterocolitis or death. J Perinatol 2009;29: 57–62.
11. Lucas A, Cole TJ. Breast milk and neonatal necrotizing enterocolitis. Lancet 1990; 336:1519–23.
12. Sisk PM, Dillard RG, Gruber KJ, et al. Early human milk feeding is associated with a lower risk of necrotizing enterocolitis in very low birth weight infants. J Perinatol 2007;27:428–33.
13. Corpeleijn WE, Kouwenhoven SM, Paap MC, et al. Intake of own mother's milk during the first days of life is associated with decreased morbidity and mortality in very low birth weight infants during the first 60 days of life. Neonatology 2012; 102:276–81.

14. Maffei D, Schanler RJ. Human milk is the feeding strategy to prevent necrotizing enterocolitis! Semin Perinatol 2017;41:36–40.

15. Rodriguez NA, Caplan MS. Oropharyngeal administration of mother's milk to prevent necrotizing enterocolitis in extremely low birth weight infants: theoretical perspectives. J Perinat Neonatal Nurs 2015;29:81–90.

16. Bocci V, von Bremen K, Corradeschi F, et al. What is the role of cytokines in human colostrum? J Biol Regul Homeost Agents 1991;5:121–4.

17. Lewis ED, Richard C, Larsen BM, et al. The importance of human milk for immunity in preterm infants [review]. Clin Perinatol 2017;44:23–47.

18. Ballard O, Morrow AL. Human milk composition, nutrients and bioactive factors. Pediatr Clin North Am 2013;60:49–74.

19. Underwood MA, Gilbert WM, Sherman MP. Amniotic fluid: not just fetal urine anymore. J Perinatol 2005;25:341–8.

20. Castellote C, Casillas R, Ramirez-Santana C, et al. Premature delivery influences the immunological composition of colostrum and transitional and mature human milk. J Nutr 2011;141:1181–7.

21. Moles L, Manzano S, Fernandez L, et al. Bacteriological, biochemical and immunological properties of colostrum and mature milk from mothers of extremely premature infants. J Pediatr Gastroenterol Nutr 2015;60:120–6.

22. Hsu Y, Chen C, Lin M, et al. Changes in preterm breast milk nutrient content in the first month. Pediatr Neonatol 2014;55:449–54.

23. Tovoy MG, Meritet JF, Guymarho J, et al. Mucosal cytokine therapy: marked antiviral and antitumor activity. J Interferon Cytokine Res 1999;19:911–21.

24. Hirai C, Ichiba H, Saito M, et al. Trophic effect of multiple growth factors in amniotic fluid or human milk on cultured human fetal small intestinal cells. J Pediatr Gastroenterol Nutr 2002;34:524–8.

25. Sullivan SE, Calhoun DA, Maheshwari A, et al. Tolerance of simulated amniotic fluid in premature neonates. Ann Pharmacother 2002;36:1518–24.

26. Donovan SM, Comstock SS. Human milk oligosaccharides influence neonatal mucosal and systemic immunity [review]. Ann Nutr Metab 2016;69(Suppl 2): 42–51.

27. Sharma D, Shastri S, Sharma P. Role of lactoferrin in neonatal care: a systematic review. J Matern Fetal Neonatal Med 2017;30:1920–32.

28. Rodriguez N, Meier P, Groer M, et al. Oropharyngeal administration of colostrum to extremely low birth weight infants: theoretical perspectives. J Perinatol 2009; 29(1):1–7.

29. Rodriguez NA, Meier PP, Groer M, et al. A pilot study to determine the safety and feasibility of oropharyngeal administration of own mother's colostrum to extremely low birth weight infants. Adv Neonatal Care 2010;10:206–12.

30. Montgomery DP, Baer VL, Lambert DK, et al. Oropharyngeal administration of colostrum to very low birth weight infants: results of a feasibility trial. Neonatal Intensive Care 2010;23:27–9, 58.

31. Rodriguez NA, Groer MW, Zeller JM, et al. A randomized controlled trial of the oropharyngeal administration of mother's colostrum to extremely low birth weight infants in the first days of life. Neonatal Intensive Care: The Journal of Perinatology-Neonatology 2011;24:31–5.

32. Martín Álvarez E, Jiménez Cabanillas MV, Peña Caballero M, et al. Efectos de la administración de calostro orofaríngeo en recién nacidos prematuros sobre los niveles de inmunoglobulina A. Nutr Hosp 2016;33:232–8.

33. Lee J, Kim HS, Jung YH, et al. Oropharyngeal colostrum administration in extremely premature infants: an RCT. Pediatrics 2015;135:e357–66.

34. Glass KM, Greecher CP, Doheny KK. Oropharyngeal administration of colostrum increases salivary secretory IgA levels in very low birth weight infants. Am J Perinatol 2017;34:1389–95.
35. Zhang Y, Ji F, Hu X, et al. Oropharyngeal colostrum administration in very low birth weight infants: a randomized controlled trial. Pediatr Crit Care Med 2017; 18:869–75.
36. Romano-Keeler J, Azcarate-Peril M, Weitkamp JH, et al. Oral colostrum priming shortens hospitalization without changing the immune-microbial milieu. J Perinatol 2017;37:36–41.
37. Sohn K, Kalanetra KM, Mills DA, et al. Buccal administration of human colostrum: impact on the oral microbiota of premature infants. J Perinatol 2016;36:106–11.
38. Seigel JK, Smith B, Ashley P, et al. Early administration of oropharyngeal colostrum to extremely low birthweight infants. Breastfeed Med 2013;8:491–5.
39. Snyder R, Herdt A, Mejias-Cepeda N, et al. Early provision of oropharyngeal colostrum leads to sustained breast milk feedings in preterm infants. Pediatr Neonatol 2017;58:534–40.
40. Rodriguez N, Vento M, Claud EC, et al. Oropharyngeal administration of mother's colostrum: health outcomes of premature infants: study protocol for a randomized controlled trial. Trials 2015;16:453.
41. Dvorak B, Fituch CC, Williams CS, et al. Increased epidermal growth factor levels in human milk of mothers with extremely premature infants. Pediatr Res 2003; 54(1):15–9.
42. Underwood M, Scoble J. Human milk and the premature infant: focus on the use of pasteurized donor human milk in the NICU. In: Rajendra R, Preedy V, Patel V, editors. Diet and nutrition in critical care. New York: Springer-Verlag; 2015. p. 795–806.
43. Picaud JC, Buffin R, Gremmo-Feger G, et al, Working Group of the French Neonatal Society on Fresh Human Milk Use in Preterm Infants. Review concludes that specific recommendations are needed to harmonise the provision of fresh mother's milk to their preterm infants. Acta Paediatr 2018;107(7):1145–55.
44. Landers S, Updegrove K. Bacteriological screening of donor human milk before and after Holder pasteurization. Breastfeed Med 2010;5:117–21.
45. Schanler R, Fraley J, Lau C, et al. Breastmilk culture and infection in extremely premature infants. J Perinatol 2011;31:335–8.
46. Bullen JJ, Rogers HJ, Leigh L. Iron-binding proteins in milk and resistance to Escherichia coli infection in infants. Br Med J 1972;1:69–75.
47. Campos LF, Domingues Repka JC, Falcão MC. Effects of human milk fortifier with iron on the bacteriostatic properties of breast milk. [[Efeitos do aditivo do leite materno com ferro sobre as propriedades bacteriostáticas do leite materno]]. J Pediatr (Rio J) 2013;89:394–9.
48. Edwards TM, Spatz DL. An innovative model for achieving breast-feeding success in infants with complex surgical anomalies. J Perinat Neonatal Nurs 2010; 24:246–53.
49. Spatz DL, Schmidt KJ. Breastfeeding success in infants with giant omphalocele. Adv Neonatal Care 2012;12:329–35.
50. Spatz DL. Innovations in the provision of human milk and breastfeeding for infants requiring intensive care. J Obstet Gynecol Neonatal Nurs 2012;41:138–43.

Does Surgical Management Alter Outcome in Necrotizing Enterocolitis?

Benjamin D. Carr, MD, Samir K. Gadepalli, MD, MBA*

KEYWORDS

- Necrotizing enterocolitis • Surgery • Metabolic derangement • Enterostomy
- Primary anastomosis • Peritoneal drainage • Laparotomy • Complications

KEY POINTS

- Surgical intervention is required in 30% to 50% of NEC cases, and carries a 40% to 50% mortality risk, with up to 70% morbidity.
- Preoperative management, surgical patient selection, and operative timing vary widely across surgeons and institutions.
- The question of peritoneal drainage versus laparotomy as both primary and definitive therapy has been investigated in two randomized controlled trials, but controversy remains.
- Surgical NEC is associated with long-term neurodevelopmental impairment, and the effect of surgical intervention remains to be established.
- The literature is dominated by retrospective cohort studies, and the future of surgical care of NEC depends on multicenter collaboration for centralized data and tissue sharing, and coordination of randomized controlled trials.

INTRODUCTION

Surgeons have been operating for necrotizing enterocolitis (NEC) since the 1940s, when it was a mysterious clinical entity known as "malignant enteritis." It was not until the 1960s that the term "necrotizing enterocolitis" was used to define "a syndrome consisting of vomiting, abdominal distention, gastrointestinal bleeding, and shock."[1,2] Since then, the principles of surgical management have not changed dramatically.[3,4] Despite the high morbidity and mortality of surgical NEC, the literature has been driven largely by nonrandomized retrospective studies until recent years, and many questions and controversies persist because of the difficulty of conducting randomized controlled trials.[5] Nevertheless, a range of surgical options exists in response to varying degrees of intestinal necrosis and systemic illness, and it is becoming clear that

Section of Pediatric Surgery, Department of Surgery, C.S. Mott Children's Hospital, University of Michigan, 1540 East Hospital Drive, SPC 4211, Ann Arbor, MI 48108, USA
* Corresponding author.
E-mail address: samirg@med.umich.edu

Clin Perinatol 46 (2019) 89–100
https://doi.org/10.1016/j.clp.2018.09.008
0095-5108/19/© 2018 Elsevier Inc. All rights reserved.

short- and long-term outcomes are affected by the choices made in the operating room and the intensive care unit. The role of primary peritoneal drainage (PD) in management of NEC has been the major surgical question of the past two decades, but other current issues include preoperative management, indications for surgery and patient selection, primary anastomosis versus enterostomy, innovative strategies for diffuse intestinal gangrene, and long-term outcomes. The future of surgical NEC research depends on collaborative efforts to standardize treatment pathways, create shared data and tissue repositories, and carefully design multicenter prospective randomized controlled trials.

SIGNIFICANCE OF SURGICAL NECROTIZING ENTEROCOLITIS

Although the overall incidence of NEC is approximately 1 in 1000 live births, incidence is 14% in infants weighing less than 1000 g, and is increasing as neonatal care for premature infants improves.[6–8] Most cases are managed medically, but 30% to 50% of infants with NEC require surgical intervention.[3,6,7,9–11] The distinction between "medical NEC" and "surgical NEC" is significant. Surgical NEC carries a mortality risk of 40% to 50%,[6,8,10,12,13] and a high morbidity in the postoperative period, with reported complication rates of 40% to 70%.[13–15] Long-term parenteral nutrition dependence occurs in 10% to 40%.[13,16,17] Stricture occurs in 10% to 35% of cases,[13,14,18,19] and dehiscence, abscess, and enterocutaneous fistula are reported at a rate of approximately 5% each.[13,20] Other complications include NEC recurrence, short gut syndrome, liver hemorrhage, hernia, and enterostomy complications.[3,13,14,21,22] Additionally, surgical NEC has been associated in numerous studies with long-term neurodevelopmental impairment (NDI).[16,23–26] Enterostomy formation as part of surgical management of NEC has also been associated with NDI, although a causal mechanism is not understood.[21] Overall, immediate postoperative outcomes have changed little in the past 30 years despite significant advances in neonatal care, whereas the long-term effects of the disease and perioperative management are only beginning to be defined. Numerous questions concerning the optimal management of surgical NEC remain unanswered.

PREOPERATIVE MANAGEMENT AND DECISION FOR SURGERY
Preoperative Management

Management of NEC is determined by the severity of disease, defined by the modified Bell staging criteria.[4,6,14,27] Most centers have developed management protocols based on Bell staging, but these protocols are idiosyncratic and no algorithmic standard exists across institutions. The tenets of medical therapy are bowel rest and decompression, intravenous fluids and nutrition, antibiotics, and serial examinations and radiographs.[4,6,14,22] However, there is wide variation in antibiotic choice and duration, even within individual centers.[22,28]

Decision for Surgery

The indications for surgery are somewhat more widely agreed on. The only absolute indication for surgical intervention is the presence of pneumoperitoneum, although some authors include clinical deterioration despite maximal medical therapy, or positive paracentesis.[3,4,10,11,22,29] Relative indications for surgery abound, and the timing and specific factors that influence the decision for surgery are widely variable.[30–33] Portal venous gas, acidosis, and precipitous thrombocytopenia are particularly ominous signs, but other relative indications include extensive pneumatosis, abdominal wall erythema, a fixed and dilated bowel loop, abdominal tenderness, greenish discoloration of the inguinal regions, and a gasless abdomen.[3,4,11,18,22,29] Notably, pneumoperitoneum is only present in approximately half of infants with perforation, making it difficult to confidently determine the ideal time to operate.[3,22] European clinicians use ultrasound as an adjunct in about half of cases, although ultrasound imaging is not standard in the United States.[32,33] Abdominal near-infrared spectroscopy is also being studied, but has not come into accepted clinical use.[3]

Several authors have pointed out that the ideal window for surgical intervention would be after irreversible bowel compromise has occurred (gangrene), but before perforation.[3,4] To this end, numerous approaches have been investigated to predict or detect NEC before severe disease, and to optimize the timing of surgery. Many surgeons use well-known biomarkers, such as platelet count, C-reactive protein, and leukocyte count, to aid in decision-making.[32,33] Several other biomarkers are under investigation, such as interleukin-8, claudin-3, inter-α inhibitor protein, fecal calprotectin, and urinary intestinal fatty acid binding protein, but none are routinely used in clinical practice.[3,10,18] The degree of systemic illness also affects surgical options and timing, and outcomes may depend more on the severity of physiologic derangement than on the surgical intervention.[31,34,35] The most widely known simple measure of metabolic derangement is the seven-item scale introduced by Tepas and colleagues,[35] who argue that the degree of metabolic derangement should determine the timing of surgery and the choice between laparotomy and PD.

PRINCIPLES OF SURGERY FOR NECROTIZING ENTEROCOLITIS

Although the spectrum of surgical options is broad, the operative strategies share common underlying goals. There are four main principles of surgical management of NEC:

- Early intervention to reduce contamination and sepsis
- Resect or defunctionalize gangrenous bowel
- Avoid or reduce multiorgan dysfunction
- Preserve bowel length to avoid short gut syndrome

The specific approach is dictated by three factors:

- Size of the infant
- Extent of disease
- Degree of metabolic derangement

Within this context, however, there is wide variation in practice patterns across surgeons and institutions.[3,4,11,18,22,29,31–33,35]

SURGICAL OPTIONS

The available surgical options depend on the extent of disease, usually classified as focal (single segment of disease), multifocal (multiple segments of disease), or panintestinal (disease affects 75% of bowel or more).[11,22] Because the extent of disease is not usually known before operation, Pierro and colleagues[36] have advocated the use of laparoscopy in the intensive care unit to guide decision-making, but this approach has not been widely adopted.[33] For focal disease, the standard operation has historically been laparotomy with resection of affected bowel followed by enterostomy, although primary anastomosis has gained acceptance in cases where the infant is physiologically stable.[22,29] This strategy can be applied to more than one segment of bowel, but in severe multifocal disease, or panintestinal disease, more advanced maneuvers may be required. Used in cases where simple resection of all affected bowel would result in short gut syndrome, these can include a high diverting jejunostomy; the "clip and drop" method with relook laparotomy; or the "patch, drain, and wait" method.[4,11,22,29] One group has even reported autoanastomosis of numerous bowel segments over an intraluminal tube.[37] In cases where the infant is deemed too physiologically unstable for laparotomy, PD is the primary temporizing option to gain control of abdominal sepsis.[17,38] Since Ein and colleagues[39] reported recovery after PD without laparotomy in a subset of patients, numerous studies have compared PD and laparotomy as both initial therapies and definitive therapies for NEC, a topic that remains controversial.

MANAGEMENT AT LAPAROTOMY

At laparotomy, the full extent of disease is assessed and necrotic bowel is resected. Classically, distal bowel is defunctionalized with formation of an enterostomy, because of concern that primary anastomosis is too high-risk in the setting of metabolic derangement and systemic inflammation. However, enterostomy also carries risks of fluid and electrolyte imbalances, skin breakdown, stoma prolapse or retraction, and the need for stoma reversal, with an overall complication rate higher than 50%.[4,14,22] Additionally, enterostomy has been associated with poorer long-term neurodevelopmental outcomes, although in a small nonrandomized retrospective study.[21] Given the complications associated with stoma formation, primary anastomosis has attracted attention as a potentially safer, simpler option. Several retrospective studies have compared enterostomy and primary anastomosis, and found that outcomes were similar in terms of morbidity and mortality, even for infants less than 1000 g.[40–42] Thus, most surgeons now perform primary anastomosis for lower-risk patients (focal disease in a larger infant), and performing enterostomy for high-risk patients (multifocal disease in smaller infants).[31,33] However, the evidence for or against primary anastomosis remains sparse, and decision-making is driven by clinical judgment.[43]

LAPAROTOMY VERSUS PERITONEAL DRAINAGE AS PRIMARY OPERATION

In the 1970s, Ein and colleagues[44] reported the bedside insertion of a peritoneal drain under local anesthesia for five infants whose low weight, prematurity, and severe metabolic derangement made them too high risk for laparotomy. This strategy gained traction over the ensuing decades, although it is not in universal use (15% to 95% of surgeons use PD, depending on the practice context).[31–33] Dozens of retrospective studies over the past three decades have reported variable results; some showed comparable survival between PD and laparotomy,[39,45–47] some showed higher mortality in the PD group,[48–50] and others posited that severity of disease and metabolic derangement determined outcome.[34,35] Over the past 20 years, several systematic reviews, meta-analyses, and prospective multicenter cohort studies have indicated that PD is associated with increased mortality,[9,12,13,51,52] with the exception of a propensity-matched Kids Inpatient Database study that showed a 47% survival with PD compared with 37% survival with laparotomy as initial treatment.[53] However, selection bias and confounding variables in most studies made it impossible to determine the effect of the primary surgical intervention, because most patients undergoing PD had more severe illness. Additionally, the understanding of spontaneous intestinal perforation (SIP) as a separate disease process from NEC has evolved during this period, and many studies included patients with both NEC and SIP. It now seems that SIP and NEC are likely distinct clinical entities, and that surgeons are able to distinguish the two preoperatively with relative confidence.[10,13,49,54–57]

Randomized Controlled Trials

Only two randomized controlled trials have addressed the question of PD versus laparotomy. The NECSTEPS trial was published in 2006 and included 117 infants with a standardized postoperative management pathway,[17] whereas the NET trial was published in 2008 and included 69 infants with discretionary postoperative management.[38] Neither trial demonstrated a significant difference in morbidity or mortality between the PD and laparotomy groups,[17,38] a conclusion further supported by a subsequent Cochrane review of both studies.[8] However, a striking difference between the two trials was the rate of salvage laparotomy after PD.[58] Previous nonrandomized studies consistently reported an early salvage laparotomy rate after PD of approximately 30%.[9,13,51,53,59] However, only five patients (9%) in the NECSTEPS trial underwent salvage laparotomy, whereas 26 patients (74%) underwent salvage laparotomy after PD in the NET trial. Rees and colleagues[60] analyzed data from the NET trial in a subsequent report to examine whether clinical status of neonates improved in the first day after PD. Comparing immediate preoperative status with 1-day postoperation in the PD group, they found no difference in organ failure score or any other measure of clinical instability. They also found no difference between preoperative and postoperative state in the laparotomy group, implying that the clinical benefit of any surgical intervention may not become apparent within the first 24 hours. The role of salvage laparotomy after PD, therefore, remains to be clarified.

Influence of Metabolic Derangement

Neither randomized trial stratified patients by degree of metabolic derangement. In a retrospective study, Tepas and colleagues[35] reported that in cases with minimal metabolic derangement, survival was higher with PD, whereas in the context of severe metabolic derangement, survival was higher with laparotomy. This implies that as a sepsis control strategy, PD may be insufficient in cases of severe disease and systemic illness, whereas in cases of mild systemic illness, the stress of laparotomy may actually contribute to physiologic decline, but this question has not been answered yet. Ehrlich and colleagues[34] have also suggested that systemic illness, not only surgical intervention, determines outcomes. Overall, despite decades of research and dozens of studies, there remains equipoise on the use of PD as the primary surgical intervention.

LAPAROTOMY VERSUS PERITONEAL DRAINAGE AS DEFINITIVE THERAPY

The use of PD as definitive therapy was introduced in a retrospective series by Ein and colleagues[39] in 1990, which reported that 32% of patients undergoing primary PD recovered without requiring laparotomy. Since then, other studies have shown that 30% to 70% of patients can be treated with PD alone.[9,10,13,51,53,59,61] Even in cases of clinical deterioration after PD, several authors have questioned the benefit of laparotomy in rescuing such patients.[17,61,62] However, not all studies distinguish between early laparotomy because of clinical decline after PD, and late laparotomy for obstruction or stricture. There is also no standardized measure of systemic illness after PD. Thus, the literature does not offer a clear picture of which patients are likely to benefit from early salvage laparotomy, and management after PD is largely based on the clinical judgment of the treating team.

Early Salvage Laparotomy in Randomized Controlled Trials

The NET and NECSTEPS trials offer disparate perspectives on this question. In the NET trial, the rate of salvage laparotomy after PD was 74%, the highest reported in the literature to date. The decision for laparotomy was at the discretion of the treating physicians, and most were performed either for persistent pneumoperitoneum and peritonitis, or signs of worsening organ function. Only 4 of 35 patients (11%) who underwent PD recovered without laparotomy (definitive therapy).[38] In the NECSTEPS trial, the rate of salvage laparotomy after PD was only 9%, because of a standardized postoperative care pathway and the study authors' perspective that "the condition of patients surviving after peritoneal drainage often deteriorates before it improves and that performing 'salvage laparotomy' after peritoneal drainage does not improve the outcome."[17] In this trial, 32 of 55 patients (58%) who underwent PD recovered without laparotomy (definitive therapy). Neither trial demonstrated a mortality benefit with laparotomy, and it seems likely that the difference in salvage laparotomy rates is more reflective of the authors' surgical paradigm than the patients' clinical state. However, the high rate of success in the NECSTEPS trial suggests that PD can serve as definitive therapy, and that an aggressive approach to early salvage laparotomy may not be necessary in all patients.

Importance of Patient Selection by Surgeons

Significantly, in the cohort of eligible but nonenrolled patients, the mortality rate for PD was comparable with the randomized cohort (41% vs 35%, respectively), whereas the mortality rate for laparotomy outperformed the randomized cohort by a large margin (15% vs 36%, respectively). As other authors have suggested, this indicates that there may be important patient selection factors that influence the success of each surgical strategy.[58] Careful patient selection by the surgeon, based on metabolic derangement and other factors, may be the key to optimal decision-making when considering laparotomy or PD for a particular patient. Studies that stratify patients by degree of systemic illness are needed to clarify this issue.

PANINTESTINAL DISEASE

Multifocal disease is found in about 55% of patients undergoing laparotomy, whereas panintestinal disease occurs in approximately 15%.[19,42,63] Outcomes in cases of severe multifocal or panintestinal disease are poor. The risk of death in panintestinal disease, defined as less than 25% of total bowel remaining, is 70% or worse, and survivors are likely to have short gut syndrome and numerous ensuing complications.[19,42,63] To preserve all possible bowel length, resection of necrotic-appearing bowel is limited or avoided altogether, and several advanced salvage strategies may be used. A high diverting jejunostomy may be used to defunctionalize distal bowel until an interval laparotomy, when resection and anastomosis can be performed.[64] A proximal enterostomy can pose difficult challenges in fluid and electrolyte management, however, and infants often require extended parenteral nutrition.[22,29] The "clip and drop" method involves resection of multiple segments of necrotic bowel, with the ends controlled using clips or stapling devices. At a second laparotomy 48 to 72 hours later, any necrotic bowel is resected. The process can then be repeated, or enteral continuity may be restored.[65] In the "patch, drain, and wait" technique, no resection is performed. Instead, sites of perforation are suture reapproximated, bilateral peritoneal drains are placed, and a decompressive gastrostomy tube is inserted. The infant then remains on extended parenteral nutrition, with the expectation that leaks and fistulas may occur, to be managed nonoperatively.[66] In some cases, the complete necrosis of bowel may be so extensive that the abdomen is simply closed, and goals of care are redirected.[19,22]

POSTOPERATIVE MANAGEMENT AND RECOVERY

Whether PD or laparotomy is undertaken, the overall clinical condition of the patient does not usually improve immediately.[60] In fact, a systemic inflammatory response is expected postoperatively, and infants may require aggressive ventilatory and circulatory support and blood product transfusion. After clinical stabilization is achieved, aggressive support measures are weaned and enteral feeds are slowly advanced. The major early complications after surgical management of NEC are stricture, abscess, dehiscence and wound healing problems, and recurrent disease. Enterostomies, if present, are generally reversed after 4 to 8 weeks. Because stricture occurs at a rate of 10% to 30%, a distal contrast study is recommended before reversal of any enterostomy. A distal stricture must also be ruled out in any case of enterocutaneous fistula, which otherwise may be expected to close with nonoperative management.[20,22,29]

Major long-term sequelae include short gut syndrome and NDI. Short gut syndrome occurs in 9% to 23% of infants with surgical NEC,[19,67] and confers long-term risks of malnutrition, chronic central access, and cholestatic liver disease.[22] NEC confers approximately 45% risk of NDI by 18 to 22 months of age,[16,24] and surgical NEC survivors are at even higher risk.[24] To date, only one nonrandomized prospective study has investigated the effect of surgical intervention on NDI, finding that PD was associated with 63% NDI in survivors, whereas laparotomy was associated with 38% NDI. There were significant differences in the PD and laparotomy groups, however, and no randomized controlled trials have reported long-term neurodevelopmental outcomes.[16] A randomized study addressing this question is scheduled to complete accrual this year.

SUMMARY: RESOLVING THE CONTROVERSIES AND MOVING FORWARD

NEC is a complex problem, and treatment has historically been driven by retrospective experience at the surgeon or institutional level. Thus, controversies remain despite decades of experience, and include the spectrum of preoperative management, indications for surgery and patient selection, PD versus laparotomy, primary anastomosis versus enterostomy, innovative strategies for panintestinal disease, and long-term outcomes. In particular, it is important to appropriately measure and consider the severity of metabolic derangement in decision-making, and to establish the role of early salvage laparotomy after PD. To resolve such questions, cooperation across institutions is necessary. Studies must carefully differentiate between SIP and NEC. Preoperative management pathways must be agreed on, and consensus on the indications for surgery must be clarified. The use of standardized biomarkers and metabolic derangement scores may facilitate diagnosis and classification of the underlying disease and the degree of systemic illness, allowing clinicians to discover which therapies are appropriate for which patients. The ideal path forward will see the creation of a national NEC registry in association with a biorepository, for shared collection and management of high-quality clinical data and tissue samples. Meanwhile, progress depends on collaborative efforts to plan and execute multicenter prospective randomized controlled trials to resolve the pressing questions faced by clinicians and families caring for infants with NEC.

Best practices

What is the current practice?

Surgical NEC

Principles of surgical management:

- Early intervention to reduce contamination and sepsis
- Resect or defunctionalize gangrenous bowel
- Avoid or reduce multiorgan dysfunction
- Preserve bowel length to avoid short gut syndrome

Specific approach determined by:

- Size of the infant
- Extent of disease
- Degree of metabolic derangement

There is wide variation in practice patterns across surgeons and institutions.

What changes in current practice are likely to improve outcomes?

- Differentiation between SIP and NEC.
- Standardized preoperative management pathways.
- Increased consideration of primary anastomosis when feasible.
- Careful patient selection for PD and laparotomy, with attention to metabolic derangement and other clinical factors.

Major Recommendations

- Multicenter collaboratives are necessary to conduct high-quality randomized controlled trials.
- A centralized NEC registry for data and tissue sharing should be established.
- Novel biomarkers and imaging techniques should be validated and integrated into clinical practice.
- Preoperative management pathways and indications for surgery should be standardized.
- Metabolic derangement should be considered when reporting outcomes of surgical interventions.
- Long-term outcomes should be reported, including NDI

REFERENCES

1. Mizrahi A, Barlow O, Berdon W, et al. Necrotizing enterocolitis in premature infants. J Pediatr 1965;66:697–706.
2. Nguyen H, Lund CH. Exploratory laparotomy or peritoneal drain? Management of bowel perforation in the neonatal intensive care unit. J Perinat Neonatal Nurs 2007;21:50–60 [quiz: 61–2].
3. Robinson JR, Rellinger EJ, Hatch LD, et al. Surgical necrotizing enterocolitis. Semin Perinatol 2017;41:70–9.
4. Henry MC, Lawrence Moss R. Surgical therapy for necrotizing enterocolitis: bringing evidence to the bedside. Semin Pediatr Surg 2005;14:181–90.
5. Hall NJ, Eaton S, Pierro A. The evidence base for neonatal surgery. Early Hum Dev 2009;85:713–8.

6. Dominguez KM, Moss RL. Necrotizing enterocolitis. Clin Perinatol 2012;39: 387–401.
7. Rees CM, Eaton S, Pierro A. National prospective surveillance study of necrotizing enterocolitis in neonatal intensive care units. J Pediatr Surg 2010;45: 1391–7.
8. Rao SC, Basani L, Simmer K, et al. Peritoneal drainage versus laparotomy as initial surgical treatment for perforated necrotizing enterocolitis or spontaneous intestinal perforation in preterm low birth weight infants. Cochrane Database Syst Rev 2011;(6):CD006182.
9. Hull MA, Fisher JG, Gutierrez IM, et al. Mortality and management of surgical necrotizing enterocolitis in very low birth weight neonates: a prospective cohort study. J Am Coll Surg 2014;218:1148–55.
10. Blakely ML, Gupta H, Lally KP. Surgical management of necrotizing enterocolitis and isolated intestinal perforation in premature neonates. Semin Perinatol 2008; 32:122–6.
11. Pierro A. The surgical management of necrotising enterocolitis. Early Hum Dev 2005;81:79–85.
12. Sola JE, Tepas JJ 3rd, Koniaris LG. Peritoneal drainage versus laparotomy for necrotizing enterocolitis and intestinal perforation: a meta-analysis. J Surg Res 2010;161:95–100.
13. Blakely ML, Lally KP, McDonald S, et al. Postoperative outcomes of extremely low birth-weight infants with necrotizing enterocolitis or isolated intestinal perforation. Ann Surg 2005;241:984–94.
14. Sato TT, Oldham KT. Abdominal drain placement versus laparotomy for necrotizing enterocolitis with perforation. Clin Perinatol 2004;31:577–89.
15. Tudehope DI. The epidemiology and pathogenesis of neonatal necrotizing enterocolitis. J Paediatr Child Health 2005;41:167–8.
16. Blakely ML, Tyson JE, Lally KP, et al. Laparotomy versus peritoneal drainage for necrotizing enterocolitis or isolated intestinal perforation in extremely low birth weight infants: outcomes through 18 months adjusted age. Pediatrics 2006; 117:e680–7.
17. Moss RL, Dimmitt RA, Barnhart DC, et al. Laparotomy versus peritoneal drainage for necrotizing enterocolitis and perforation. N Engl J Med 2006;354:2225–34.
18. Frost BL, Modi BP, Jaksic T, et al. New medical and surgical insights into neonatal necrotizing enterocolitis: a review. JAMA Pediatr 2017;171:83–8.
19. Ricketts RR, Jerles ML. Neonatal necrotizing enterocolitis: experience with 100 consecutive surgical patients. World J Surg 1990;14:600–5.
20. Stringer MD, Cave E, Puntis JW, et al. Enteric fistulas and necrotizing enterocolitis. J Pediatr Surg 1996;31:1268–71.
21. Ta BD, Roze E, van Braeckel KN, et al. Long-term neurodevelopmental impairment in neonates surgically treated for necrotizing enterocolitis: enterostomy associated with a worse outcome. Eur J Pediatr Surg 2011;21:58–64.
22. Kastenberg ZJ, Sylvester KG. The surgical management of necrotizing enterocolitis. Clin Perinatol 2013;40:135–48.
23. Hintz SR, Kendrick DE, Stoll BJ, et al. Neurodevelopmental and growth outcomes of extremely low birth weight infants after necrotizing enterocolitis. Pediatrics 2005;115:696–703.
24. Rees CM, Pierro A, Eaton S. Neurodevelopmental outcomes of neonates with medically and surgically treated necrotizing enterocolitis. Arch Dis Child Fetal Neonatal Ed 2007;92:F193–8.

25. Schulzke SM, Deshpande GC, Patole SK. Neurodevelopmental outcomes of very low-birth-weight infants with necrotizing enterocolitis: a systematic review of observational studies. Arch Pediatr Adolesc Med 2007;161:583–90.
26. Wadhawan R, Oh W, Hintz SR, et al. Neurodevelopmental outcomes of extremely low birth weight infants with spontaneous intestinal perforation or surgical necrotizing enterocolitis. J Perinatol 2014;34:64–70.
27. Neu J, Walker WA. Necrotizing enterocolitis. N Engl J Med 2011;364:255–64.
28. Blackwood BP, Hunter CJ, Grabowski J. Variability in antibiotic regimens for surgical necrotizing enterocolitis highlights the need for new guidelines. Surg Infect (Larchmt) 2017;18:215–20.
29. Thakkar HS, Lakhoo K. The surgical management of necrotising enterocolitis (NEC). Early Hum Dev 2016;97:25–8.
30. Henry MC, Moss RL. Necrotizing enterocolitis. Annu Rev Med 2009;60:111–24.
31. Rees CM, Hall NJ, Eaton S, et al. Surgical strategies for necrotising enterocolitis: a survey of practice in the United Kingdom. Arch Dis Child Fetal Neonatal Ed 2005;90:F152–5.
32. Valpacos M, Arni D, Keir A, et al. Diagnosis and management of necrotizing enterocolitis: an international survey of neonatologists and pediatric surgeons. Neonatology 2018;113:170–6.
33. Zani A, Eaton S, Puri P, et al. International survey on the management of necrotizing enterocolitis. Eur J Pediatr Surg 2015;25:27–33.
34. Ehrlich PF, Sato TT, Short BL, et al. Outcome of perforated necrotizing enterocolitis in the very low-birth weight neonate may be independent of the type of surgical treatment. Am Surg 2001;67:752–6.
35. Tepas JJ 3rd, Sharma R, Hudak ML, et al. Coming full circle: an evidence-based definition of the timing and type of surgical management of very low-birth-weight (<1000 g) infants with signs of acute intestinal perforation. J Pediatr Surg 2006; 41:418–22.
36. Pierro A, Hall N, Ade-Ajayi A, et al. Laparoscopy assists surgical decision making in infants with necrotizing enterocolitis. J Pediatr Surg 2004;39:902–6.
37. Lessin MS, Schwartz DL, Wesselhoeft CW. Multiple spontaneous small bowel anastomosis in premature infants with multisegmental necrotizing enterocolitis. J Pediatr Surg 2000;35:170–2.
38. Rees CM, Eaton S, Kiely EM, et al. Peritoneal drainage or laparotomy for neonatal bowel perforation? A randomized controlled trial. Ann Surg 2008;248:44–51.
39. Ein SH, Shandling B, Wesson D, et al. A 13-year experience with peritoneal drainage under local anesthesia for necrotizing enterocolitis perforation. J Pediatr Surg 1990;25:1034–6 [discussion: 1036–7].
40. Hall NJ, Curry J, Drake DP, et al. Resection and primary anastomosis is a valid surgical option for infants with necrotizing enterocolitis who weigh less than 1000 g. Arch Surg 2005;140:1149–51.
41. Singh M, Owen A, Gull S, et al. Surgery for intestinal perforation in preterm neonates: anastomosis vs stoma. J Pediatr Surg 2006;41:725–9 [discussion: 725–9].
42. Fasoli L, Turi RA, Spitz L, et al. Necrotizing enterocolitis: extent of disease and surgical treatment. J Pediatr Surg 1999;34:1096–9.
43. Downard CD, Renaud E, St Peter SD, et al. Treatment of necrotizing enterocolitis: an American Pediatric Surgical Association Outcomes and Clinical Trials Committee systematic review. J Pediatr Surg 2012;47:2111–22.
44. Ein SH, Marshall DG, Girvan D. Peritoneal drainage under local anesthesia for perforations from necrotizing enterocolitis. J Pediatr Surg 1977;12:963–7.

45. Azarow KS, Ein SH, Shandling B, et al. Laparotomy or drain for perforated necrotizing enterocolitis: who gets what and why? Pediatr Surg Int 1997;12:137–9.
46. Mishra P, Foley D, Purdie G, et al. Intestinal perforation in premature neonates: the need for subsequent laparotomy after placement of peritoneal drains. J Paediatr Child Health 2016;52:272–7.
47. Sharma R, Tepas JJ, Mollitt DL, et al. Surgical management of bowel perforations and outcome in very low-birth-weight infants (≤1,200 g). J Pediatr Surg 2004;39: 190–4.
48. Broekaert I, Keller T, Schulten D, et al. Peritoneal drainage in pneumoperitoneum in extremely low birth weight infants. Eur J Pediatr 2018;177:853–8.
49. Chiu B, Pillai SB, Almond PS, et al. To drain or not to drain: a single institution experience with neonatal intestinal perforation. J Perinat Med 2006;34:338–41.
50. Rakshasbhuvankar A, Rao S, Minutillo C, et al. Peritoneal drainage versus laparotomy for perforated necrotising enterocolitis or spontaneous intestinal perforation: a retrospective cohort study. J Paediatr Child Health 2012;48:228–34.
51. Choo S, Papandria D, Zhang Y, et al. Outcomes analysis after percutaneous abdominal drainage and exploratory laparotomy for necrotizing enterocolitis in 4,657 infants. Pediatr Surg Int 2011;27:747–53.
52. Moss RL, Dimmitt RA, Henry MC, et al. A meta-analysis of peritoneal drainage versus laparotomy for perforated necrotizing enterocolitis. J Pediatr Surg 2001; 36:1210–3.
53. Tashiro J, Wagenaar AE, Perez EA, et al. Peritoneal drainage is associated with higher survival rates for necrotizing enterocolitis in premature, extremely low birth weight infants. J Surg Res 2017;218:132–8.
54. Hwang H, Murphy JJ, Gow KW, et al. Are localized intestinal perforations distinct from necrotizing enterocolitis? J Pediatr Surg 2003;38:763–7.
55. Okuyama H, Kubota A, Oue T, et al. A comparison of the clinical presentation and outcome of focal intestinal perforation and necrotizing enterocolitis in very-low-birth-weight neonates. Pediatr Surg Int 2002;18:704–6.
56. Pumberger W, Mayr M, Kohlhauser C, et al. Spontaneous localized intestinal perforation in very-low-birth-weight infants: a distinct clinical entity different from necrotizing enterocolitis. J Am Coll Surg 2002;195:796–803.
57. Tarrado X, Castanon M, Thio M, et al. Comparative study between isolated intestinal perforation and necrotizing enterocolitis. Eur J Pediatr Surg 2005;15:88–94.
58. Raval MV, Hall NJ, Pierro A, et al. Evidence-based prevention and surgical treatment of necrotizing enterocolitis-a review of randomized controlled trials. Semin Pediatr Surg 2013;22:117–21.
59. Demestre X, Ginovart G, Figueras-Aloy J, et al. Peritoneal drainage as primary management in necrotizing enterocolitis: a prospective study. J Pediatr Surg 2002;37:1534–9.
60. Rees CM, Eaton S, Khoo AK, et al. Peritoneal drainage does not stabilize extremely low birth weight infants with perforated bowel: data from the NET Trial. J Pediatr Surg 2010;45:324–8 [discussion: 328–9].
61. Morgan LJ, Shochat SJ, Hartman GE. Peritoneal drainage as primary management of perforated NEC in the very low birth weight infant. J Pediatr Surg 1994;29:310–5.
62. Dimmitt RA, Meier AH, Skarsgard ED, et al. Salvage laparotomy for failure of peritoneal drainage in necrotizing enterocolitis in infants with extremely low birth weight. J Pediatr Surg 2000;35:856–9.
63. Voss M, Moore SW, van der Merwe I, et al. Fulminating necrotising enterocolitis: outcome and prognostic factors. Pediatr Surg Int 1998;13:576–80.

64. Thyoka M, Eaton S, Kiely EM, et al. Outcomes of diverting jejunostomy for severe necrotizing enterocolitis. J Pediatr Surg 2011;46:1041–4.
65. Vaughan WG, Grosfeld JL, West K, et al. Avoidance of stomas and delayed anastomosis for bowel necrosis: the 'Clip and drop-back' technique. J Pediatr Surg 1996;31:542–5.
66. Moore TC. Successful use of the "patch, drain, and wait" laparotomy approach to perforated necrotizing enterocolitis: is hypoxia-triggered "good angiogenesis" involved? Pediatr Surg Int 2000;16:356–63.
67. Horwitz JR, Lally KP, Cheu HW, et al. Complications after surgical intervention for necrotizing enterocolitis: a multicenter review. J Pediatr Surg 1995;30:994–9.

Epidemiology of Necrotizing Enterocolitis

New Considerations Regarding the Influence of Red Blood Cell Transfusions and Anemia

Vivek Saroha, MD, PhD[a], Cassandra D. Josephson, MD[b,c],
Ravi Mangal Patel, MD, MSc[a,*]

KEYWORDS

- Infant • Neonate • Preterm • Blood • Oxygenation • Morbidity

KEY POINTS

- The optimal hemoglobin thresholds to administer red blood cell (RBC) transfusion are currently uncertain.
- Results of ongoing randomized trials are likely to provide important new evidence to guide RBC transfusion.
- Until new trial data are available, it is advisable to avoid using routine RBC transfusion thresholds above the liberal arm or below the conservative arm of thresholds studied in trials to date in preterm infants, as the safety of such approaches is uncertain.
- Practices to minimize RBC transfusion and anemia, such as placental transfusion by delayed cord clamping, have important benefits but it is unclear if these practices reduce NEC.

Conflicts of Interest: Dr C.D. Josephson has received oxygenation monitoring equipment (eg, NIRS and pulse oximetry) from Medtronic, Inc. The company had no role in this review. The other authors have no conflicts of interest to report.
The review was supported, in part, by the National Institutes of Health under award K23 HL128942 (R.M. Patel), which had no role in the content of this review.
[a] Division of Neonatal-Perinatal Medicine, Department of Pediatrics, Emory University School of Medicine, Children's Healthcare of Atlanta, 2015 Uppergate Drive Northeast, 3rd Floor, Atlanta, GA 30322, USA; [b] Center for Transfusion and Cellular Therapies, Department of Pathology and Laboratory Medicine, Emory University School of Medicine, 101 Woodruff Circle, Atlanta, GA 30322, USA; [c] Department of Pediatrics, Emory University School of Medicine, 101 Woodruff Circle, Atlanta, GA 30322, USA
* Corresponding author.
E-mail address: rmpatel@emory.edu

Clin Perinatol 46 (2019) 101–117
https://doi.org/10.1016/j.clp.2018.09.006
0095-5108/19/© 2018 Elsevier Inc. All rights reserved.

INTRODUCTION

Necrotizing enterocolitis (NEC) is major contributor to morbidity and mortality in infants, accounting for 10% of deaths in the neonatal intensive care unit.[1,2] Recent data suggest the incidence of NEC is decreasing in the United States[3]; however, the reported incidence of NEC is highly variable among high-income countries.[4] The pathogenesis of NEC is multifactorial and includes innate, maternal, and postnatal risk factors. Multiple observational studies have demonstrated an association between NEC and the potentially modifiable risk factors of anemia and red blood cell (RBC) transfusion. Some investigators have proposed that the occurrence of NEC in temporal association with an RBC transfusion is a distinct clinical entity, separate from non–transfusion-associated NEC.[5] This review appraises data on the epidemiology of NEC with a focus on the potential role of RBC transfusion and anemia.

OVERVIEW OF TRANSFUSION PRACTICES

Neonatal hemoglobin (Hb) levels decline in the days and weeks after birth.[6] Preterm infants, in comparison with term infants, have a relatively lower Hb level at birth[7] and experience a greater Hb decline during the neonatal period.[8] This decline in Hb often leads to treatment with an RBC transfusion. The ideal threshold for administering an RBC transfusion is currently not known. Clinicians often consider the Hb level along with the postnatal age of the infant and need for cardiorespiratory support to guide their decision for when to administer an RBC transfusion. Studies of direct comparisons of restrictive (low Hb threshold) versus liberal (high Hb threshold) strategies are limited to 3 randomized controlled trials[9–11] and 2 ongoing trials.[12,13] The Hb transfusion thresholds in the restrictive and liberal arms of these trials are summarized in **Table 1**.

Temporal trends suggest increasingly restrictive RBC transfusion practices, with acceptance of a lower concentration of Hb before an RBC transfusion.[14–16] In the absence of a clear advantage of either approach, the optimal Hb transfusion threshold remains uncertain with a recent Cochrane review justifying clinical equipoise.[17]

DATA ON RED BLOOD CELL TRANSFUSION AND NECROTIZING ENTEROCOLITIS

Since the publication of several initial reports of a temporal association between RBC transfusion and NEC,[18–20] multiple subsequent observational studies[21–36] have reported on the association between RBC transfusion and NEC. Most of these observational studies report on NEC occurring within 48 hours of an RBC transfusion, although the 48-hour cutoff is arbitrary.

Several systematic reviews and meta-analyses have summarized and evaluated the potential association between RBC transfusion and NEC (**Table 2**). Two meta-analyses of observational studies[37,38] were published in 2017. A meta-analysis by Garg and colleagues[37] of 17 observational studies reported no evidence of an association between exposure to RBC transfusion and the risk of NEC (odds ratio [OR] 0.96, 95% confidence interval [CI] 0.53–1.71, $P = .88$) with high study heterogeneity ($I^2 = 93\%$). In addition, the investigators performed subgroup analyses and found heterogeneity in results by study type (cohort studies and case-control studies). Analysis of data from 4 cohort studies showed a significant association between RBC transfusion and a lower risk of NEC (OR 0.51, 95% CI 0.34–0.75, $P = <.01$) with low statistical heterogeneity ($I^2 = 28\%$). By comparison, subgroup analysis of 13 case-control studies showed no difference in odds for NEC with RBC transfusion (OR 1.20, 95% CI 0.58–2.47, $P = .63$) with high heterogeneity ($I^2 = 93\%$). Another meta-analysis by

Table 1
Hemoglobin transfusion thresholds used in clinical trials

Study	Postnatal Age, d	Clinical Status	Restrictive Hb Threshold, g/dL[a]	Liberal Hb Threshold, g/dL[a]
PINT trial,[10] 2005	1–7	Any respiratory support (capillary/central sample)	11.5/10.4	13.5/12.2
		No respiratory support (capillary/central sample)	10.0/9.0	12.0/10.9
	8–14	Any respiratory support (capillary/central sample)	10.0/9.0	12.0/10.9
		No respiratory support (capillary/central sample)	8.5/7.7	10.0/9.0
	≥15	Any respiratory support (capillary/central sample)	8.5/7.7	10.0/9.0
		No respiratory support (capillary/central sample)	7.5/6.8	8.5/7.7
Bell et al,[9] 2005		Ventilated	11.3	15.3
		CPAP or oxygen	9.3	12.7
		No respiratory support	7.3	10.0
Chen et al,[11] 2009		Ventilated	11.7	15.0
		CPAP	10.0	13.3
		Spontaneous breathing	7.3	10.0
TOP trial[12]	Week 1	Any respiratory support	11.0	13.0
		No respiratory support	10.0	12.0
	Week 2	Any respiratory support	10.0	12.5
		No respiratory support	8.5	11.0
	Week 3	Any respiratory support	8.5	11.0
		No respiratory support	7.0	10.0
ETTNO trial[13]	3–7	Critical[b]	11.3	13.6
		Noncritical[b]	9.3	11.7
	8–21	Critical[b]	10.0	12.3
		Noncritical[b]	8.0	10.3
	>21	Critical[b]	9.0	11.3
		Noncritical	7.0	9.3

Abbreviations: CPAP, continuous positive airway pressure; ETTNO, Effects of Transfusion Thresholds on Neurocognitive Outcome of Extremely Low Birth Weight Infants; Hb, hemoglobin; PINT, Premature Infants in Need of Transfusion; TOP, Transfusion of Prematurity.

[a] If hematocrit was reported, the Hb threshold was approximated by dividing by 3.

[b] Critical defined as any of the following: (1) requirement of mechanical ventilation, (2) requirement of CPAP with FiO_2 greater than 0.25 for more than 12 hours per 24 hours, (3) patent ductus arteriosus requiring therapy, (4) more than 6 apneas that require stimulation per 24 hours, or more than 4 desaturations to SpO_2 less than 60% per 24 hours despite methylxanthines and CPAP, and (5) acute sepsis or acute necrotizing enterocolitis requiring inotropic or vasopressor support.

Table 2
Meta-analyses of observational studies reporting on RBC transfusion and NEC

Study Author, Year	Number of Studies	Study Types	NEC Events Related to RBC Transfusion/Total	NEC Events Unrelated to RBC Transfusion/Total	I², %	Summary Odds Ratio (95% CI)
Kirpalani & Zupancic,[40] 2012	6	Cohort studies	150/2940	192/19,215	98	7.48 (5.87–9.53)
	4	Case-control studies	129/186	129/381	92	2.19 (1.52–3.17)
Mohamed & Shah,[39] 2012	5	All observational studies reporting unadjusted estimates	N/A	N/A	58	3.91 (2.97–5.14)
	4	All observational studies reporting adjusted estimates	N/A	N/A	91	2.01 (1.61–2.50)
Garg et al,[37] 2017	17	All observational studies	N/A	N/A	93	0.96 (0.53–1.71)
	4	Cohort studies	N/A	N/A	28	0.51 (0.34–0.75)
	13	Case-control studies (3 unmatched, 10 matched)	N/A	N/A	93	1.20 (0.58–2.47)
Hay et al,[38] 2017	13	All observational studies reporting on NEC within 48 h of transfusion	479/4498	1242/7104	93	1.13 (0.99–1.29)
	9	All observational studies reporting on NEC at any time after transfusion	334/2380	256/2541	86	1.95 (1.60–2.38)

Abbreviations: CI, confidence interval; N/A, not available; NEC, necrotizing enterocolitis; RBC, red blood cell.

Hay and colleagues[38] of 13 observational studies found no evidence of an association between RBC transfusion and NEC occurring within 48 hours of transfusion (OR 1.13, 95% CI 0.99–1.29) with high statistical heterogeneity among studies (I^2 = 93%). The investigators concluded that there was a very low confidence of a true relationship between RBC transfusion and NEC, based on the Grading of Recommendations Assessment, Development, and Evaluation (GRADE) system.

These results from more recent meta-analyses are in contrast to results of 2 previous meta-analyses of observational studies in 2012 by Mohamed and Shah[39] and by Kirpalani and Zupancic[40] that reported an increased risk of NEC within 48 hours after receiving an RBC transfusion. The meta-analysis by Mohamed and Shah[39] of 4 studies reported a pooled adjusted OR for NEC of 2.01 (95% CI 1.61–2.50, I^2 = 91%) among RBC-exposed infants. Kirpalani and Zupancic[40] included only full-length publications and excluded data from abstracts and reported an increased risk for NEC with blood transfusion in 6 cohort studies (unadjusted OR 7.48, CI 5.87–9.53) and in 4 case-control studies (OR 2.19, CI 1.52–3.17).

The differences in the results of meta-analyses from 2012 and 2017 may be from publication bias, as noted by Hay and colleagues,[38] with earlier studies predominantly reporting positive associations between RBC transfusion and NEC and more recent studies reporting no association and some suggesting RBC transfusion may be protective toward NEC. In addition, a meta-analysis of randomized trials[40] comparing restrictive and liberal transfusion strategies in preterm infants found no effect of more restrictive thresholds (leading to fewer RBC transfusions), compared with liberal RBC transfusion thresholds (leading to more RBC transfusions) on the risk of NEC (OR 1.67, 95% CI 0.82–3.38). Notably, the estimates are heavily weighted by a single trial (PINT trial)[10] with weight of 89% (**Table 3**). In addition, these trials did not report on a temporal relationship between RBC transfusion and NEC. In the absence of higher-quality data, the question of does RBC transfusion cause NEC remains unresolved.

DATA ON ANEMIA AND NECROTIZING ENTEROCOLITIS

Several observational studies that reported on an association between RBC transfusion and NEC did not report a significant effect of anemia as an independent risk for NEC.[23,24,29,41] However, in a case-control study, Singh and colleagues[30] identified 111 preterm (≤32 weeks) infants with NEC and 222 matched controls and reported that, after controlling for other factors, each 1-point decrease in the nadir hematocrit was associated with a 10% increase in odds for NEC (OR 1.10, 95% CI 1.02–1.18). Patel and colleagues,[42] in a prospective multicenter study, reported that in a given week, severe anemia, defined as Hb level of 8.0 g/dL or less, was associated with a higher adjusted risk for NEC (adjusted cause-specific hazard ratio 5.99, 95% CI

Study Author, Year	Number of Trials	NEC Events with Restrictive RBC Transfusion Threshold	NEC Events with Liberal RBC Transfusion Threshold	I^2	Odd Ratio of NEC (95% CI), Restrictive vs Liberal RBC Transfusion Threshold
Table 3 Meta-analyses of randomized trials reporting on RBC transfusion and NEC					
Kirpalani & Zupancic,[40] 2012	3	21/292	13/298	0%	1.67 (0.82–3.38)

Note: Estimates similar to meta-analyses by Whyte and Kirpalani[17] and, therefore, not repeated.
Abbreviations: CI, confidence interval; NEC, necrotizing enterocolitis; RBC, red blood cell.

2.00–18.0, $P = .001$); however, the study did not evaluate the interaction between severe anemia and RBC transfusion. A recent case-crossover study by Le and colleagues,[43] designed to identify an association of NEC with RBC transfusion, feed advances, or fortification, found no evidence of an association between RBC transfusion and NEC (OR 1.80, 95% CI 0.60–5.37). A subgroup analysis showed that among anemic infants (Hb ≤9.3 g/dL), the risk of RBC transfusion on NEC was higher (OR 6; 95% CI 0.72–49.8) compared with those without anemia (OR 1, 95% CI 0.20–4.95), but the difference in effect estimates among subgroups was not statistically significant.

It is plausible that the occurrence of NEC after an RBC transfusion is the result of interaction between the effect of anemia and the effect of RBC transfusion. Evaluating such an interplay between the contribution of anemia and RBC transfusion is challenging in clinical studies, as assessing interaction between 2 exposures (anemia and RBC transfusion) typically requires a much larger sample size than assessing the effect of a single exposure (anemia or RBC transfusion). In addition, lower Hb oxygen saturation targeting, an important determinant of oxygenation that increases the risk of NEC,[44] has not been measured, controlled, or reported in observational studies of RBC transfusion-associated NEC, limiting the understanding of the interaction between Hb saturation and anemia. Preclinical studies offer an opportunity to assess the biologic plausibility of such an interaction and may provide data on the potential of such an interaction that is challenging to assess without very large, adequately powered randomized trials. Two ongoing, large randomized trials[12,13] comparing liberal and restrictive transfusion thresholds are designed to assess the effect of high versus low transfusion thresholds on survival and long-term neurocognitive outcomes; however, with NEC as a secondary outcome measure, these trials may contribute important data on the effect of both RBC transfusion and anemia (by comparing high and low Hb transfusion thresholds) on NEC when these results are considered alongside those of prior trials.

POTENTIAL MECHANISMS UNDERLYING THE ASSOCIATIONS

The development of NEC in an infant is considered the final common endpoint of a multitude of etiologic pathways[45] that result in disruption of mucosal integrity and inflammation from responses to intraluminal pathogenic organisms. Several mechanisms for intestinal injury in response to RBC transfusion, with or without the presence of anemia, have been proposed (**Fig. 1**) and are discussed in additional detail in the following section.

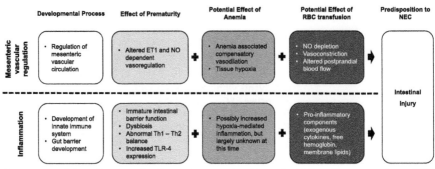

Fig. 1. Potential mechanisms for the pathogenesis of intestinal injury from anemia and RBC transfusion. ET1, endothelin 1; NO, nitric oxide; Th, T helper cell; TLR-4, toll-like receptor 4.

Hypoxemia and Dysregulation of Mesenteric Blood Flow

Reversible binding of oxygen to Hb accounts for more than 98% of oxygen carriage by blood. At physiologic partial pressure of oxygen, 100 mL of plasma contains 0.3 mL of oxygen. In comparison, each gram of Hb can combine with 1.34 mL of oxygen.[46] A decrease in blood Hb concentration leads to circulatory adjustments, such as increases in capillary perfusion and increased oxygen extraction by tissues.[46,47] However, worsening anemia may overwhelm the compensatory mechanisms and significantly impair the ability of blood to meet oxygen demands of the tissues causing hypoxia,[48] which may be worsened in the setting of lower oxygen saturation targets.[44] Molecular compensatory mechanisms exist to maintain the gut barrier in the setting of hypoxia[49,50]; however, it has been proposed that progressive hypoxia may reach a critical imbalance in oxygen delivery as compared with consumption, leading to mucosal barrier injury[51] and poor mucosal healing,[52] predisposing the neonate to development of NEC.[5]

In a growing neonate, the intestines proliferate as the gut elongates and the mucosa grows. Active expression of angiogenic factors in the metabolically active and rapidly proliferating gut mucosa ensures concomitant development of vascular structures in the intestine.[53] It has been proposed that the developing thin arterioles may be structurally weak, and on exposure to an RBC transfusion and associated alterations in oxygen availability, blood pressure, flow, or viscosity, these arterioles are prone to injury, precipitating ischemic injury to the gut mucosa.[5,54] However, experimental evidence is needed to confirm the proposed mechanisms.

Mesenteric or splanchnic blood flow is determined by a dynamic balance between vasoconstrictive and vasodilatory inputs by mediators such as endothelin-1 (ET-1) and nitric oxide (NO).[54] Ontogeny of the regulatory mechanisms of the mesenteric vascular tone during the neonatal period demonstrates distinct responses to autonomic, humoral, and paracrine factors as compared with a mature infant.[55,56] In the newborn, the balance is favored toward NO-mediated vasodilation.[55,57] In addition, as compared with older subjects, NO inhibition leads to a greater increase in vascular resistance in newborn animal models.[58–60] RBC transfusion leads to an alteration in postprandial response to mesenteric blood flow as evident from a clinical study by Krimmel and colleagues.[61] Analysis of preprandial and postprandial mesenteric blood flow in 22 infants (mean gestational age, 27.3 weeks, mean postmenstrual age, 31.8 weeks) demonstrated that anemia was associated with increased flow in the superior mesenteric artery following feeding, which was evident pre-transfusion and absent in the immediate post-transfusion state. One potential mechanism for this decreased blood flow is by RBC transfusion–associated depletion of intravascular NO.[62] This may be secondary to depletion of NO in RBCs during storage, consumption of NO through binding to free Hb released from hemolysis, or from release of arginase from RBCs, which depletes the NO precursor arginine.[62] The transient anemia-associated hypoxia followed by reperfusion after RBC transfusion and associated dysregulation of blood flow may have a cumulative and/or interactive role in pathogenesis of disease.[63]

Role of Inflammation

The occurrence of NEC in response to RBC transfusion or anemia has been proposed to be the outcome of a 2-hit mechanism,[5] similar to the proposed mechanisms for transfusion-related acute lung injury (TRALI), a condition that can occur following transfusion of any blood component. In TRALI, underlying clinical conditions lead to endothelial activation in the host (first hit), which in the presence of a blood product transfusion and associated exposure to mediators, such as donor HLA antibodies, biologically active lipids, free Hb, red cell membrane fragments, and inflammatory cytokines (second hit), leads to a severe inflammatory response and associated lung injury.

It has been proposed that the immature neonatal gut is in a heightened state of immune activation and prone to inflammation. Multiple factors, such as mucosal exposure to substrates, hypoxia, and changes in the gut microbiome associated with the use of antibiotics and formula feeds,[5,16,64–66] have been proposed to contribute to inflammation and associated phenotypic shift of T helper (T_H) cells from T_H2 to T_H1.[67] Upregulation of Toll-Like Receptors (TLRs), particularly TLR-4,[68] is a significant contributor to intestinal inflammation.[68,69]

In such a background, RBC transfusion can potentially introduce biological response modifiers such as donor antibodies,[70] cytokines in stored blood,[71] free Hb,[72] lipids from RBC membranes, and white cells generating an exaggerated systemic immune response that may cause gut mucosal inflammation and injury. Dani and colleagues[73] demonstrated serum cytokine changes after an RBC transfusion event in 20 infants of less than 32 weeks' gestational age. The study identified significant increases in interferon-gamma, monocyte chemoattractant protein-1, intracellular adhesion molecule-1, and interleukin (IL)-1β, IL-8, and IL-17 after an RBC transfusion. Ho and colleagues[74] measured fecal calprotectin (FC) before and after 46 RBC transfusion events in 26 very low birthweight (VLBW) infants, and showed that FC was higher than baseline after RBC transfusion and was higher in multiply-transfused infants. Notably, FC was the highest in infants with the lowest pretransfusion hematocrits and in those who received RBCs that had been stored for more than 21 days.

In a background of constitutive vasodilation and increased reactivity in the neonatal gut vasculature, despite compensatory hemodynamic and molecular changes, progressive anemia may reach a critical level leading to hypoxia. RBC transfusion in such a state may lead to depletion of NO and loss of vasodilation along with abnormal regulation of mesenteric blood flow leading to tissue ischemic injury. Multiple factors associated with prematurity such as dysbiosis and increased TLR-4 expression cause a state of inflammation in the intestinal mucosa that can potentially increase with hypoxia. Introduction of exogenous biological response modifiers in transfused products may lead to heightened immune responses leading to damage to the intestinal mucosa. However, additional data are needed from both human and preclinical studies to better understand the mechanisms that may underlie the possible adverse effects of both RBC transfusion and anemia on the neonatal intestine.

INFLUENCE OF CLINICAL STRATEGIES TO PREVENT ANEMIA AND RED BLOOD CELL TRANSFUSION

Iatrogenic phlebotomy loss, a result of intensive clinical monitoring in critically ill newborns, is a major cause of neonatal anemia and driver of RBC transfusion.[75] The common strategies to minimize blood sampling in the neonatal intensive care unit include the use of noninvasive monitoring and point of care testing[76] and use of umbilical cord blood for admission blood tests for VLBW preterm neonates.[77] With a combination of several approaches and ongoing vigilance, studies have shown a significant effect in preventing anemia and decreasing RBC transfusion.[78]

Placental transfusion achieved by delayed clamping of the umbilical cord after birth or by milking of the umbilical cord before clamping is now recommended as standard care for neonatal resuscitation of preterm infants.[79–81] A 2012 Cochrane review of 15 randomized controlled trials, 5 of which reported NEC as an outcome measure, indicated a decreased risk for NEC in infants receiving delayed cord clamping, compared with immediate cord clamping (n = 241, RR 0.62, 95% CI 0.43–0.9).[82] However, a more recent meta-analysis, including 12 studies that reported on NEC, found that delayed cord clamping was not associated with a decreased risk for NEC for all infants less than 37 weeks' gestation at birth (n = 2397, RR 0.88, CI 0.65–1.18) and for infants born <28 weeks' gestation (4 studies, n = 977, RR 0.87, CI 0.61–1.24).[83] The quality of evidence was determined as low using the GRADE criteria. Notably, the findings of this recent meta-analysis were weighted heavily by the Australian Placental Transfusion Study of 1566 infants born at less than 30 weeks' gestation, randomized to placental transfusion by delayed cord clamping or early clamping.[84] In this trial 44 (6.2%) of 712 infants randomized to delayed cord clamping developed NEC, as compared with 41 infants (5.6%) of 734 randomized to early clamping. Importantly, the effect of delayed cord clamping on Hb nadir and RBC transfusion requirements is likely to depend on postnatal RBC transfusion approaches.

Apart from its role in prompting erythropoiesis and decreasing need for RBC transfusion, erythropoietin (EPO), which is also present in breast milk,[85] may play a role in intestinal development, cellular repair,[86] and inhibition of NO formation.[87] Ledbetter and Juul[88] first reported an association of recombinant human erythropoietin (rEPO) administration in infants ≤1250 g and a decreased incidence of NEC (4.6% in the rEPO group as compared with 10% in controls). A recent Cochrane meta-analysis of a randomized controlled trial of early (age <8 days) administration of erythropoiesis-stimulating agents (ESAs) (EPO or darbepoietin) versus placebo or no intervention included 15 studies (n = 2639).[89] The analysis demonstrated a significantly reduced risk for NEC (any stage) in the ESA group compared with the placebo group (RR 0.69, 95% CI 0.52–0.91, I^2 = 0%). The quality of the evidence was deemed moderate.[89,90] Previous concerns regarding the increased risk for retinopathy of prematurity (all stages) with EPO administration[91] were not demonstrated in this meta-analysis (11 studies, n = 2185, RR 0.92, 95% CI 0.79–1.08; I^2 = 0%).[89,91] A Cochrane meta-analysis of late EPO administration (8–28 days) in extremely low birthweight infants (6 studies, n = 656) did not demonstrate any difference in the risk for NEC with EPO as compared with placebo or no intervention (RR 0.88, 95% CI 0.46–1.69, I^2 = 0%).[90] Late EPO was associated with a nonsignificant trend toward an increased risk for retinopathy of prematurity (ROP) (stage ≥3, 3 studies, n = 442) with an RR 1.73 (95% CI 0.92–3.24, I^2 = 18%) and for all ROP stages (3 studies, n = 404) with an RR 1.27 (95% CI 0.99–1.64, I^2 = 83%). Two ongoing large randomized trials of EPO administration in preterm infants, Preterm Erythropoietin Neuroprotection Trial (PENUT Trial, NCT01378273)[92] and Erythropoietin in Premature Infants to Prevent Encephalopathy (NCT02550054), include NEC as a secondary outcome and will provide additional evidence regarding the effect of EPO on the risk of NEC and the safety of EPO administration in different populations.

ROLE OF FEEDING DURING RED BLOOD CELL TRANSFUSION

With the recognition of a potential association between RBC transfusion and development of NEC, there has been interest in withholding feeding during RBC transfusion. In prospective observational studies, feeding immediately after RBC transfusion has been associated with an attenuation of the postprandial increase in superior mesenteric artery blood flow velocity as compared with the pretransfusion measurements made using pulse Doppler ultrasound.[61,93] However, a prospective observational comparison of infants less than 33 weeks at birth who were fed (n = 9) or not fed (n = 8) during RBC transfusion demonstrated that mesenteric tissue oxygenation, as measured by using near-infrared spectroscopy (NIRS), was not influenced by feeding.[94]

A systematic review of 7 observational studies reported that withholding feeds during RBC transfusion was associated with lower risk of NEC associated with transfusion (n = 7492, RR 0.47, 95% CI 0.28–0.80, I^2 = 11%).[95] Although biologically plausible, the results from these observational studies remain vulnerable to bias and confounding. A large randomized controlled trial, Withholding Enteral Feeds Around Transfusion (WHEAT) trial is currently under way[96] and will hopefully provide evidence to answer the clinically relevant question of whether feeding during an RBC transfusion causes NEC.

ROLE OF NEAR-INFRARED SPECTROSCOPY

NIRS is a noninvasive technique for monitoring regional tissue oxygenation in real time. NIRS measures the difference between oxyHb and deoxyHb, which reflects oxygen uptake in the specific tissue bed measured.[97] This measurement, which is reported as the regional oxygen saturation (rSO_2), reflects the balance of oxygen that is delivered minus what is extracted at the tissue level.[97] A decreasing NIRS rSO_2 reading indicates either increasing oxygen extraction at the tissue level or decreasing oxygen delivery to tissues in the region measured.

With its ability to monitor mesenteric tissue oxygenation,[98] use of NIRS to monitor intestinal oxygenation in preterm infants has been studied.[99] Bailey and colleagues[100] demonstrated large variability of mesenteric oxygenation during RBC transfusion in preterm neonates. Marin and colleagues[101] compared NIRS measurements in 4 patients with NEC associated with RBC transfusion with 4 controls who received RBC transfusion but did not develop NEC. This study demonstrated wide fluctuation and decreases in mesenteric oxygenation patterns that were more pronounced in infants who developed NEC with RBC transfusion as compared with non-NEC infants. In a pilot study, Sood and colleagues[102] compared the mesenteric and cerebral rSO_2 patterns of infants who did not develop NEC within 7 days of RBC transfusion (n = 120), infants who developed NEC within 7 days before RBC transfusion (n = 20), and infants who developed NEC within 7 days after an RBC transfusion (n = 8). The study reported decreases in mesenteric rSO_2 during and after an RBC transfusion in infants who went on to develop NEC within 7 days as compared with the other 2 groups that had an increase in rSO_2.

Although promising, there is currently no evidence to support the use of NIRS monitoring to guide RBC transfusion approaches to prevent NEC. Two prospective trials registered at clinicaltrials.gov, Transfusion of Prematurity (TOP trial) NCT01702805 and Combining Restrictive Guidelines and an NIRS SCORE to Decrease RBC Transfusions, include NIRS monitoring at different thresholds for RBC transfusion. The data from these trials may provide more insight into the utility of this technique into identifying the need for RBC transfusion and allow for a better understanding of the effects of RBC transfusion and anemia on intestinal oxygenation and NEC.

SUMMARY

Observational studies have provided conflicting evidence regarding the effect of RBC transfusion and anemia on NEC. It is possible that anemia and/or RBC transfusion may lead to tissue hypoxia, dysregulation of mesenteric vascular regulation, or inflammation. Such mechanisms may act independently or in combination to lead to intestinal injury and, potentially, the development of NEC. Placental transfusion and the use of

ESA have a role in decreasing RBC transfusion and anemia, although it is unclear if these treatments reduce NEC. Ongoing RBC transfusion trials have the potential to provide additional evidence to improve our understanding of transfusion strategies to decrease the risk for NEC.

Best practices

What is the current practice?

Currently, there is uncertainty regarding the optimal Hb thresholds to transfuse RBCs into preterm infants.

What changes in current practice are likely to improve outcomes?

The following practices are suggested:

1. Provide placental transfusion, when feasible.

2. Minimize unnecessary phlebotomy-related blood losses.

3. Avoid using routine RBC transfusion thresholds above the liberal Hb level or below the conservative Hb level of thresholds studied to date, as the safety of such approaches is uncertain.

Summary Statement

Results of data from 2 multicenter randomized trials of high versus low transfusion thresholds (TOP, ETTNO) are likely to provide important new evidence to guide RBC transfusion. Until these data are available, no confident conclusions regarding the effects of RBC transfusion or anemia on NEC can currently be provided.

REFERENCES

1. Stoll BJ, Hansen NI, Bell EF, et al. Trends in care practices, morbidity, and mortality of extremely preterm neonates, 1993-2012. JAMA 2015;314(10):1039–51.
2. Jacob J, Kamitsuka M, Clark RH, et al. Etiologies of NICU deaths. Pediatrics 2015;135(1):e59–65.
3. Horbar JD, Edwards EM, Greenberg LT, et al. Variation in performance of neonatal intensive care units in the United States. JAMA Pediatr 2017;171(3): e164396.
4. Battersby C, Santhalingam T, Costeloe K, et al. Incidence of neonatal necrotising enterocolitis in high-income countries: a systematic review. Arch Dis Child Fetal Neonatal Ed 2018;103(2):F182–9.
5. La Gamma EF, Blau J. Transfusion-related acute gut injury: feeding, flora, flow, and barrier defense. Semin Perinatol 2012;36(4):294–305.
6. Lundstrom U, Siimes MA, Dallman PR. At what age does iron supplementation become necessary in low-birth-weight infants? J Pediatr 1977;91(6):878–83.
7. Blanchette VS, Zipursky A. Assessment of anemia in newborn infants. Clin Perinatol 1984;11(2):489–510.
8. Widness JA. Pathophysiology of anemia during the neonatal period, including anemia of prematurity. Neoreviews 2008;9(11):e520.
9. Bell EF, Strauss RG, Widness JA, et al. Randomized trial of liberal versus restrictive guidelines for red blood cell transfusion in preterm infants. Pediatrics 2005; 115(6):1685–91.
10. Kirpalani H, Whyte RK, Andersen C, et al. The Premature Infants in Need of Transfusion (PINT) study: a randomized, controlled trial of a restrictive (low)

versus liberal (high) transfusion threshold for extremely low birth weight infants. J Pediatr 2006;149(3):301–7.

11. Chen HL, Tseng HI, Lu CC, et al. Effect of blood transfusions on the outcome of very low body weight preterm infants under two different transfusion criteria. Pediatr Neonatal 2009;50(3):110–6.

12. Kirpalani H, Bell EF, D'Angio C, et al. Transfusion of prematures (TOP) trial: does a liberal red blood cell transfusion strategy improve neurologically-intact survival of extremely-low-birth-weight infants as compared to a restrictive strategy? NICHD Neonatal Research Network; 2016. Available at: https://www.nichd.nih.gov/sites/default/files/about/Documents/TOP_Protocol.pdf. Accessed May 20, 2018.

13. Investigators E. The 'effects of transfusion thresholds on neurocognitive outcome of extremely low birth-weight infants (ETTNO)' study: background, aims, and study protocol. Neonatology 2012;101(4):301–5.

14. Maier RF, Sonntag J, Walka MM, et al. Changing practices of red blood cell transfusions in infants with birth weights less than 1000 g. J Pediatr 2000; 136(2):220–4.

15. Ekhaguere OA, Morriss FH Jr, Bell EF, et al. Predictive factors and practice trends in red blood cell transfusions for very-low-birth-weight infants. Pediatr Res 2016;79(5):736–41.

16. Guidelines for transfusion of erythrocytes to neonates and premature infants. Fetus and Newborn Committee, Canadian Paediatric Society. CMAJ 1992; 147(12):1781–92.

17. Whyte R, Kirpalani H. Low versus high haemoglobin concentration threshold for blood transfusion for preventing morbidity and mortality in very low birth weight infants. Cochrane Database Syst Rev 2011;(11):CD000512.

18. McGrady GA, Rettig PJ, Istre GR, et al. An outbreak of necrotizing enterocolitis. Association with transfusions of packed red blood cells. Am J Epidemiol 1987; 126(6):1165–72.

19. Agwu JC, Narchi H. In a preterm infant, does blood transfusion increase the risk of necrotizing enterocolitis? Arch Dis Child 2005;90(1):102–3.

20. Short A, Gallagher A, Ahmed M. Necrotizing enterocolitis following blood transfusion. Electronic letter to the Editor. Arch Dis Child. 2005 Apr 14. Available at: https://adc.bmj.com/content/90/1/102.responses.

21. Mally P, Golombek SG, Mishra R, et al. Association of necrotizing enterocolitis with elective packed red blood cell transfusions in stable, growing, premature neonates. Am J Perinatol 2006;23(8):451–8.

22. Holder G, Doherty D, Patole S. Elective red cell transfusions for anemia of prematurity and development of necrotizing enterocolitis in previously well preterm neonates: incidence and difficulties in proving a cause-effect relation. J Neonatal Perinatal Med 2009;2(3):181–6.

23. Christensen RD, Lambert DK, Henry E, et al. Is "transfusion-associated necrotizing enterocolitis" an authentic pathogenic entity? Transfusion 2010;50(5): 1106–12.

24. Josephson CD, Wesolowski A, Bao G, et al. Do red cell transfusions increase the risk of necrotizing enterocolitis in premature infants? J Pediatr 2010;157(6): 972–8.e1-3.

25. Blau J, Calo JM, Dozor D, et al. Transfusion-related acute gut injury: necrotizing enterocolitis in very low birth weight neonates after packed red blood cell transfusion. J Pediatr 2011;158(3):403–9.

26. Couselo M, Aguar M, Ibáñez V, et al. Relation between packed red blood cell transfusion and severity of necrotizing enterocolitis in premature infants. Cir Pediatr 2011;24(3):137–41 [in Spanish].

27. El-Dib M, Narang S, Lee E, et al. Red blood cell transfusion, feeding and necrotizing enterocolitis in preterm infants. J Perinatol 2011;31(3):183–7.

28. Ghirardello S, Lonati CA, Dusi E, et al. Necrotizing enterocolitis and red blood cell transfusion. J Pediatr 2011;159(2):354–5.

29. Paul DA, Mackley A, Novitsky A, et al. Increased odds of necrotizing enterocolitis after transfusion of red blood cells in premature infants. Pediatrics 2011; 127(4):635–41.

30. Singh R, Visintainer PF, Frantz ID 3rd, et al. Association of necrotizing enterocolitis with anemia and packed red blood cell transfusions in preterm infants. J Perinatol 2011;31(3):176–82.

31. Carter BM, Holditch-Davis D, Tanaka D, et al. Relationship of neonatal treatments with the development of necrotizing enterocolitis in preterm infants. Nurs Res 2012;61(2):96–102.

32. Stritzke AI, Smyth J, Synnes A, et al. Transfusion-associated necrotising enterocolitis in neonates. Arch Dis Child Fetal Neonatal Ed 2013;98(1):F10–4.

33. Wan-Huen P, Bateman D, Shapiro DM, et al. Packed red blood cell transfusion is an independent risk factor for necrotizing enterocolitis in premature infants. J Perinatol 2013;33(10):786–90.

34. AlFaleh K, Al-Jebreen A, Baqays A, et al. Association of packed red blood cell transfusion and necrotizing enterocolitis in very low birth weight infants. J Neonatal Perinatal Med 2014;7(3):193–8.

35. Baxi AC, Josephson CD, Iannucci GJ, et al. Necrotizing enterocolitis in infants with congenital heart disease: the role of red blood cell transfusions. Pediatr Cardiol 2014;35(6):1024–9.

36. Garg PM, Ravisankar S, Bian H, et al. Relationship between packed red blood cell transfusion and severe form of necrotizing enterocolitis: a case control study. Indian Pediatr 2015;52(12):1041–5.

37. Garg P, Pinotti R, Lal CV, et al. Transfusion-associated necrotizing enterocolitis in preterm infants: an updated meta-analysis of observational data. J Perinat Med 2018;46(6):677–85.

38. Hay S, Zupancic JAF, Flannery DD, et al. Should we believe in transfusion-associated enterocolitis? Applying a GRADE to the literature. Semin Perinatol 2017;41(1):80–91.

39. Mohamed A, Shah PS. Transfusion associated necrotizing enterocolitis: a meta-analysis of observational data. Pediatrics 2012;129(3):529–40.

40. Kirpalani H, Zupancic JA. Do transfusions cause necrotizing enterocolitis? The complementary role of randomized trials and observational studies. Semin Perinatol 2012;36(4):269–76.

41. Wallenstein MB, Arain YH, Birnie KL, et al. Red blood cell transfusion is not associated with necrotizing enterocolitis: a review of consecutive transfusions in a tertiary neonatal intensive care unit. J Pediatr 2014;165(4):678–82.

42. Patel RM, Knezevic A, Shenvi N, et al. Association of red blood cell transfusion, anemia, and necrotizing enterocolitis in very low-birth-weight infants. JAMA 2016;315(9):889–97.

43. Le VT, Klebanoff MA, Talavera MM, et al. Transient effects of transfusion and feeding advances (volumetric and caloric) on necrotizing enterocolitis development: a case-crossover study. PLoS One 2017;12(6):e0179724.

44. Askie LM, Darlow BA, Finer N, et al. Association between oxygen saturation targeting and death or disability in extremely preterm infants in the neonatal oxygenation prospective meta-analysis collaboration. JAMA 2018;319(21): 2190–201.

45. Schnabl KL, Aerde JEV, Thomson ABR, et al. Necrotizing enterocolitis: a multifactorial disease with no cure. World J Gastroenterol 2008;14(14):2142–61.

46. Pittman RN. Regulation of tissue oxygenation, chapter 4, oxygen transport. San Rafael (CA): Morgan & Claypool Life Sciences; 2011.

47. Szabo JS, Mayfield SR, Oh W, et al. Postprandial gastrointestinal blood flow and oxygen consumption: effects of hypoxemia in neonatal piglets. Pediatr Res 1987;21(1):93–8.

48. Tsui AKY, Marsden PA, Mazer CD, et al. Differential HIF and NOS responses to acute anemia: defining organ-specific hemoglobin thresholds for tissue hypoxia. Am J Physiol Regul Integr Comp Physiol 2014;307(1):R13–25.

49. Furuta GT, Turner JR, Taylor CT, et al. Hypoxia-inducible factor 1-dependent induction of intestinal trefoil factor protects barrier function during hypoxia. J Exp Med 2001;193(9):1027–34.

50. Colgan SP, Curtis VF, Lanis JM, et al. Metabolic regulation of intestinal epithelial barrier during inflammation. Tissue Barriers 2015;3(1–2):e970936.

51. Lauscher PMD, Kertscho HMD, Schmidt O, et al. Determination of organ-specific anemia tolerance. Crit Care Med 2013;41(4):1037–45.

52. Schreml S, Szeimies RM, Prantl L, et al. Oxygen in acute and chronic wound healing. Br J Dermatol 2010;163(2):257–68.

53. Holmes K, Charnock Jones SD, Forhead AJ, et al. Localization and control of expression of VEGF-A and the VEGFR-2 receptor in fetal sheep intestines. Pediatr Res 2008;63(2):143–8.

54. Nowicki PT. Ischemia and necrotizing enterocolitis: where, when, and how. Semin Pediatr Surg 2005;14(3):152–8.

55. Watkins DJ, Besner GE. The role of the intestinal microcirculation in necrotizing enterocolitis. Semin Pediatr Surg 2013;22(2):83–7.

56. Nankervis CA, Giannone PJ, Reber KM. The neonatal intestinal vasculature: contributing factors to necrotizing enterocolitis. Semin Perinatol 2008;32(2): 83–91.

57. Nankervis CA, Nowicki PT. Role of nitric oxide in regulation of vascular resistance in postnatal intestine. Am J Physiol 1995;268(6 Pt 1):G949–58.

58. Nowicki PT, Nankervis CA, Miller CE. Effects of ischemia and reperfusion on intrinsic vascular regulation in the postnatal intestinal circulation. Pediatr Res 1993;33(4 Pt 1):400–4.

59. Dani C, Pratesi S, Fontanelli G, et al. Blood transfusions increase cerebral, splanchnic, and renal oxygenation in anemic preterm infants. Transfusion 2010;50(6):1220–6.

60. Bailey SM, Hendricks-Munoz KD, Wells JT, et al. Packed red blood cell transfusion increases regional cerebral and splanchnic tissue oxygen saturation in anemic symptomatic preterm infants. Am J Perinatol 2010;27(6):445–53.

61. Krimmel GA, Baker R, Yanowitz TD. Blood transfusion alters the superior mesenteric artery blood flow velocity response to feeding in premature infants. Am J Perinatol 2009;26(2):99–105.

62. Bennett-Guerrero E, Veldman TH, Doctor A, et al. Evolution of adverse changes in stored RBCs. Proc Natl Acad Sci U S A 2007;104(43):17063–8.

63. Howarth C, Banerjee J, Aladangady N. Red blood cell transfusion in preterm infants: current evidence and controversies. Neonatology 2018;114(1):7–16.

64. Hosny M, Cassir N, La Scola B. Updating on gut microbiota and its relationship with the occurrence of necrotizing enterocolitis. Human Microbiome Journal 2017;4:14–9.
65. Pammi M, Cope J, Tarr PI, et al. Intestinal dysbiosis in preterm infants preceding necrotizing enterocolitis: a systematic review and meta-analysis. Microbiome 2017;5(1):31.
66. Maheshwari A, Kelly DR, Nicola T, et al. TGF-β2 suppresses macrophage cytokine production and mucosal inflammatory responses in the developing intestine. Gastroenterology 2011;140(1):242–53.
67. Zhang B, Ohtsuka Y, Fujii T, et al. Immunological development of preterm infants in early infancy. Clin Exp Immunol 2005;140(1):92–6.
68. Lu P, Hackam DJ. Toll-like receptor regulation of intestinal development and inflammation in the pathogenesis of necrotizing enterocolitis. Pathophysiology 2014;21(1):81–93.
69. Nino DF, Sodhi CP, Hackam DJ. Necrotizing enterocolitis: new insights into pathogenesis and mechanisms. Nat Rev Gastroenterol Hepatol 2016;13(10): 590–600.
70. Wang-Rodriguez J, Fry E, Fiebig E, et al. Immune response to blood transfusion in very-low-birthweight infants. Transfusion 2000;40(1):25–34.
71. Kristiansson M, Soop M, Saraste L, et al. Cytokines in stored red blood cell concentrates: promoters of systemic inflammation and simulators of acute transfusion reactions? Acta Anaesthesiol Scand 1996;40(4):496–501.
72. Sachs UJ. Recent insights into the mechanism of transfusion-related acute lung injury. Curr Opin Hematol 2011;18(6):436–42.
73. Dani C, Poggi C, Gozzini E, et al. Red blood cell transfusions can induce proinflammatory cytokines in preterm infants. Transfusion 2017;57(5):1304–10.
74. Ho TT, Groer MW, Luciano AA, et al. Red blood cell transfusions increase fecal calprotectin levels in premature infants. J Perinatol 2015;35(10):837–41.
75. Rosebraugh MR, Widness JA, Nalbant D, et al. A mathematical modeling approach to quantify the role of phlebotomy losses and need for transfusions in neonatal anemia. Transfusion 2013;53(6):1353–60.
76. Lemyre B, Sample M, Lacaze-Masmonteil T. Minimizing blood loss and the need for transfusions in very premature infants. Paediatr Child Health 2015;20(8): 451–62.
77. Prescott A, C.R. Darnall Army Medical Center, Walter Reed National Military Medical Center, et al. Umbilical cord blood use for admission blood tests of very low birth weight preterm neonates: a multi-center randomized clinical trial. 2018. Available at: https://ClinicalTrials.gov/show/NCT02103296. Accessed May 20, 2018.
78. Rabe H, Alvarez JR, Lawn C, et al. A management guideline to reduce the frequency of blood transfusion in very-low-birth-weight infants. Am J Perinatol 2009;26(3):179–83.
79. Delayed umbilical cord clamping after birth. Pediatrics 2017;139(6) [pii: e20170957].
80. Committee opinion No. 684: delayed umbilical cord clamping after birth. Obstet Gynecol 2017;129(1):e5–10.
81. WHO Guidelines Approved by the Guidelines Review Committee. Guidelines on basic newborn resuscitation. Geneva (Switzerland): World Health Organization; 2012.
82. Rabe H, Diaz-Rossello JL, Duley L, et al. Effect of timing of umbilical cord clamping and other strategies to influence placental transfusion at preterm birth

on maternal and infant outcomes. Cochrane Database Syst Rev 2012;(8):CD003248.

83. Fogarty M, Osborn DA, Askie L, et al. Delayed vs early umbilical cord clamping for preterm infants: a systematic review and meta-analysis. Am J Obstet Gynecol 2018;218(1):1–18.

84. Tarnow-Mordi W, Morris J, Kirby A, et al. Delayed versus immediate cord clamping in preterm infants. N Engl J Med 2017;377(25):2445–55.

85. Juul SE, Joyce AE, Zhao Y, et al. Why is erythropoietin present in human milk? Studies of erythropoietin receptors on enterocytes of human and rat neonates. Pediatr Res 1999;46(3):263–8.

86. McPherson RJ, Juul SE. High-dose erythropoietin inhibits apoptosis and stimulates proliferation in neonatal rat intestine. Growth Horm IGF Res 2007;17(5): 424–30.

87. Kumral A, Baskin H, Duman N, et al. Erythropoietin protects against necrotizing enterocolitis of newborn rats by the inhibiting nitric oxide formation. Biol Neonate 2003;84(4):325–9.

88. Ledbetter DJ, Juul SE. Erythropoietin and the incidence of necrotizing enterocolitis in infants with very low birth weight. J Pediatr Surg 2000;35(2):178–81 [discussion: 182].

89. Ohlsson A, Aher SM. Early erythropoiesis-stimulating agents in preterm or low birth weight infants. Cochrane Database Syst Rev 2017;(11):CD004863.

90. Aher SM, Ohlsson A. Late erythropoietin for preventing red blood cell transfusion in preterm and/or low birth weight infants. Cochrane Database Syst Rev 2014;(4):CD004868.

91. Romagnoli C, Zecca E, Gallini F, et al. Do recombinant human erythropoietin and iron supplementation increase the risk of retinopathy of prematurity? Eur J Pediatr 2000;159(8):627–8.

92. National Institute of Neurological Disorders and Stroke. Preterm erythropoietin neuroprotection trial (PENUT trial). 2018. Available at: https://ClinicalTrials.gov/show/NCT01378273. Accessed June 8, 2018.

93. Pitzele A, Rahimi M, Armbrecht E, et al. Packed red blood cell transfusion (PRBC) attenuates intestinal blood flow responses to feedings in pre-term neonates with normalization at 24 hours. J Matern Fetal Neonatal Med 2015;28(15): 1770–3.

94. Marin T, Josephson CD, Kosmetatos N, et al. Feeding preterm infants during red blood cell transfusion is associated with a decline in postprandial mesenteric oxygenation. J Pediatr 2014;165(3):464–71.e1.

95. Jasani B, Rao S, Patole S. Withholding feeds and transfusion-associated necrotizing enterocolitis in preterm infants: a systematic review. Adv Nutr 2017;8(5): 764–9.

96. Gale C, Hyde MJ, Modi N. Research ethics committee decision-making in relation to an efficient neonatal trial. Arch Dis Child Fetal Neonatal Ed 2017;102(4): F291–8.

97. Moore JE. Newer monitoring techniques to determine the risk of necrotizing enterocolitis. Clin Perinatol 2013;40(1):125–34.

98. Fortune PM, Wagstaff M, Petros AJ. Cerebro-splanchnic oxygenation ratio (CSOR) using near infrared spectroscopy may be able to predict splanchnic ischaemia in neonates. Intensive Care Med 2001;27(8):1401–7.

99. Cortez J, Gupta M, Amaram A, et al. Noninvasive evaluation of splanchnic tissue oxygenation using near-infrared spectroscopy in preterm neonates. J Matern Fetal Neonatal Med 2011;24(4):574–82.

100. Bailey SM, Hendricks-Munoz KD, Mally PV. Variability in splanchnic tissue oxygenation during preterm red blood cell transfusion given for symptomatic anaemia may reveal a potential mechanism of transfusion-related acute gut injury. Blood Transfus 2015;13(3):429–34.
101. Marin T, Moore J, Kosmetatos N, et al. Red blood cell transfusion-related necrotizing enterocolitis in very-low-birthweight infants: a near-infrared spectroscopy investigation. Transfusion 2013;53(11):2650–8.
102. Sood BG, Cortez J, McLaughlin K, et al. Near infrared spectroscopy as a biomarker for necrotising enterocolitis following red blood cell transfusion. J Near Infrared Spectrosc 2014;22(6):375–88.

Role of Abdominal US in Diagnosis of NEC

Jae H. Kim, MD, PhD[a,b]

KEYWORDS

- Necrotizing enterocolitis • Bowel ultrasound • Pneumatosis intestinalis

KEY POINTS

- Diagnosing bowel integrity in necrotizing enterocolitis (NEC) continues to be a challenge with current clinical, laboratory, and radiographic means.
- Bowel ultrasound (BUS) can demonstrate high spatial resolution of tissue texture, blood perfusion, and peristaltic activity.
- BUS presents a novel opportunity to improve NEC diagnosis and management for surgery decision making.
- Considerable effort is required to introduce BUS into the neonatologist's algorithm for assessing NEC and for diagnostic imaging, to incorporate these new techniques into their workflow.

BACKGROUND

Necrotizing enterocolitis (NEC) is a severe gastrointestinal inflammatory condition that disrupts the physiology and tissue architecture of the gut. These changes can be evaluated by several static and dynamic imaging modalities. The development of NEC starts with scattered or diffuse transmural inflammation involving any segment of the small or large bowel. This leads to physical changes in the bowel wall beginning with dilatation of the bowel wall and thickening as blood flow and swelling increases. The affected loops may change from flattened or semifilled loops of bowel to more rigid and dilated loops of bowel. With such inflammation, intestinal motility can be affected and result in more dilatation of the affected and proximal bowel as transit slows. This transmural inflammation can also lead to weeping of fluid from the serosa into the peritoneal space. A classic feature of NEC is the mucosal invasion

Disclosure Statement: J.H. Kim is a consultant for Medela, Ferring, Alcresta. He was a past speaker for Mead Johnson and Abbott Nutrition. He owns shares in Nicolette, Pediasolutions, and Astarte Medical Partners.
[a] SPIN Program, San Diego Mothers' Milk Bank, Division of Neonatology, UC San Diego, 9300 Campus Point Drive MC7774, La Jolla, CA 92037, USA; [b] Division of Pediatric Gastroenterology, Hepatology and Nutrition, Rady Children's Hospital-San Diego, 3020 Children's Way, San Diego, CA 92123
E-mail address: neojae@ucsd.edu

with gas-forming bacteria that generate intramural gas bubbles that are identified on abdominal radiograph (ARs) as pneumatosis intestinalis. Occasionally large amounts of gas may also enter the portal venous system as well. The terminal phases of NEC involve loss of blood flow and further dilatation with thinning of the bowel wall that can ultimately can lead to bowel wall perforation. The resulting peritonitis may cause mixed ascites and particulate matter within the ascites. Each imaging modality is discussed with respect to value in diagnosing or managing NEC. The potential for bowel ultrasound (BUS) to improve diagnostic and management of bowel injury in NEC is discussed in this article.

THE LIMITATIONS OF ABDOMINAL RADIOGRAPHS

The greatest values of the plain AR are the ease and frequency of use that enable it often to be the first sign or corroborating sign of bowel pathology. An AR can demonstrate abnormal bowel patterns and can show gas-filled dilated loops of bowel, pneumatosis intestinalis or portal venous gas, and frank perforation. The paucity of gas or presence of fixed dilated loops of bowel is a suspicious sign. ARs are static and, therefore, not able to display dynamic function bowel, such as peristalsis. Large amounts of ascites may be visible because they can push the bowel loops to cluster centrally on AR. The 2 biggest weaknesses of the AR are the insensitivity in detecting bowel perforation and the difficulty in accurately diagnosing pneumatosis intestinalis. The risk of missing bowel perforation is high and may lead to greater morbidity and mortality. On the other side, the risk of overdiagnosing an AR with NEC is consequential, too. Infants diagnosed with suspected NEC could be unfed for 10 days to 14 days and started on broad-spectrum intravenous antibiotics. There is some irony in this because there is a higher risk of NEC in those infants who are exposed to longer durations of antibiotics.[1] Regardless of these limitations, there has been little practical adaptation in neonatology to evaluate bowel through imaging modalities other than AR.

THE BENEFITS OF ULTRASOUND

There have been increasing opportunities with ultrasound (US) to obtain higher resolution as well as dynamic imaging without the need for additional radiation in evaluating bowel health. The use of US continues to increase for specialized applications in medicine whether evaluation the contents of a joint or the retina of the eye. The benefits of US include the portable ease of use at the bedside; the ability to discern different tissue densities, particularly of fluid nature; the lack of ionizing radiation; and the broadening application by care providers in point-of-care management, such as in the emergency department.

A majority of applications to date with BUS have been in adult or pediatric patients and much fewer in neonatal ones. The various applications have included assessment of acute appendicitis, intussusception, bowel obstruction, and inflammatory bowel disease.[2–4] The use of BUS is increasingly helpful with patients with inflammatory bowel disease, where the hallmarks of inflammation can involve small and large intestines and partial-thickness or full-thickness bowel wall inflammation.[5] These assessments are further expanding to include refined cross-sectional assessment of bowel to better characterize inflammation with US and other modalities.[6] Also, postsurgical strictures can be assessed accurately with BUS.[7]

Emergency medicine has shown that learning to identify bowel obstruction is relatively simple and comparable to CT diagnosis.[8,9] The detection of an inflamed acute appendix as in appendicitis is a skill that emergency department physician have been able to show has value in specificity when identified and obviate other imaging. The absence of findings of an acute appendix are not conclusive and does not rule out an appendicitis, however.[10] Several studies have demonstrated that gastroesophageal reflux can be evaluated by US, both identifying anatomic risk factors and visualizing the bolus, but this has not expanded much in clinical practice yet.[11,12]

NEONATAL APPLICATIONS
Blood Flow

The superior mesenteric artery (SMA) arises from the anterior surface of the abdominal aorta and supplies the majority of the small intestine and large intestine from the lower part of the duodenum to the proximal two-thirds of the transverse colon. Therefore, the initial application of US in bowel injury and assessment was with interrogation of the SMA because it is the key blood source to the majority of the bowel and is readily visible in the upper abdomen. The visualization of the SMA is possible using either a low-frequency phase array (6–10 MHz) or high-frequency linear probe (greater than 10 MHz).

Measuring SMA flow can assist in determining large vessel flow patterns in a variety of clinical situations. The SMA flow has been shown different between bolus feeding and continuous feeding where the former and not the latter produced a rise in splanchnic blood flow.[13] Measuring SMA flow may help discern infants who are at higher risk with feeding difficulties.[14] The pulsatility index was strongly correlated with infant feeding difficulties. Others have shown that the SMA peak systolic velocity (PSV) does not seem to change significantly across gestational or with time after enteral feeding.[15] The diagnosis of intestinal malrotation with volvulus by US has been used in the past. The orientation of the SMA on the aortic axis with a potential to twist into a whirlpool sign can provide a high degree of sensitivity and specificity in making this diagnosis.[16]

Peristalsis

Current assessment of bowel motility is limited. At bedside clinical examination is depended on, which includes visual inspection, palpation, and auscultation of bowel sounds. The sensitivity and specificity of some these assessments are not reliable because abdominal distension may be present when hyperperistalsis is present, such as in bowel obstruction, or ileus, such as in sepsis. The presence of bowel sounds is subject to the presence of air-fluid interfaces in the bowel. Many loops of bowel may mostly be fluid-filled and less likely to produce audible bowel sounds. Bowel US can be used to quantify and characterize the bowel motility in the first week of life.[17] Cumulative bowel motility can be scored to demonstrate a gradual increase in bowel motility in the first 5 days of life with or without feeding. A simpler global assessment of bowel motility can also be defined by grading overall motility by being absent, low active, normoactive, or hyperactive (unpublished). More work is required to further characterize these cumulative scoring or global assessment and its value in supporting clinical decision making, particularly around feeding. More normative data are needed to determine the impact of feeding on intestinal peristalsis of the preterm infant. Identifying peristalsis offers the promise of assisting in the routine management of neonatal feeding or bowel assessment, but further studies are required to validate its utility for changing clinical outcomes.

BOWEL ULTRASOUND FOR NECROTIZING ENTEROCOLITIS

The preterm infant and term infant are ideal subjects for BUS due to their small size and the thinness of their abdominal wall. Although gas can be present in the bowel, which can obscure the view, significant portions of bowel are only fluid-filled and readily visualized. Static gray-scale BUS images reveal bowel shape, size, wall thickness and degree of dilatation, and accumulation of the bowel ascites with a high degree of accuracy (**Fig. 1**). BUS can display dynamic changes in bowel, such as peristalsis and blood perfusion. BUS has numerous aspects that make it superior to AR (**Table 1**). Intestinal peristalsis in NEC decreases with progression of disease, with greater involvement of bowel. Although the characterization of peristalsis by BUS is still undergoing quantitative and global assessment validation, simple assessment of peristalsis can begin to help discern between bowel obstruction, where there is hyperactivity, versus sepsis or NEC where hypoperistalsis is present.

Regional blood flow through the SMA has been shown to have value in the early detection of changes with infants with suspected NEC.[18–20] The SMA PSV and end-diastolic velocity were found lower in infants who develop NEC. In the study by Hashem and colleagues, few of the subjects were fed, so this may have confounded their data.[18] The celiac–to–SMA PSV ratio was significantly higher in those infants who developed NEC, supportive of regional differences in resistance in the 2 splanchnic beds supplied. Measures of resistive index or pulsatility index also may be helpful with the diagnosis of NEC.[20]

Several studies have shown that BUS is helpful in evaluating the viability of bowel in preterm infants suspected of having NEC.[21–32] In these studies, the gray-scale characteristics of bowel can be detailed. These include static physical characteristics, such as bowel wall thickness, wall diameter, dilatation, and echogenicity, as well as dynamic imaging of peristalsis and perfusion. Imaging and detecting pneumatosis intestinalis is more accurate with BUS due to the spatial resolution of the air within the bowel wall and the ability to discriminate individual gas bubbles (**Fig. 2**). With color Doppler, specific suspicious loops of bowel can be interrogated to reveal if they are perfused or not, which enables the identification of nonviable bowel with a high degree of certainty. Faingold and colleagues found that there was 100% correlation between BUS and necrotic bowel in infants with surgical NEC (**Fig. 3**).[25] The gradual progression of NEC can be described by BUS from the initial hyperemia and swelling of bowel

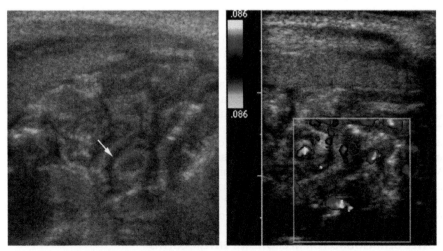

Fig. 1. Normal gray-scale image of bowel. Left panel: white arrow indicated loop of bowel. (*From* Faingold R, Daneman A, Tomlinson G, et al. Necrotizing enterocolitis: assessment of bowel viability with color Doppler US. Radiology 2005;235(2):589; with permission.)

Table 1
Comparison of specificity and sensitivity of abdominal radiographs to ultrasound

	Abdominal Radiographs		Abdominal Ultrasound	
Findings	Specificity	Sensitivity	Specificity	Sensitivity
Ascites	Low	Low	High	High
Perforation	High	Low	High	High
Bowel wall thickness	Low	Low	High	High
Bowel dilatation	High	Mid (misses fluid-filled loops)	High	High
Pneumatosis	Mid	Mid	High	High
Motility	N/A	N/A	High	High

wall to the dilatation with increased disease and then thinning of bowel wall with loss of perfusion or blood flow.[24] The detection of portal venous gas is better with BUS than by radiographs due to the high echogenic signal air produced.[33] In a direct comparison of ARs and sonograms, findings of thickened bowel wall, intramural gas, portal venous gas, and reduced peristalsis were independent risk factors for the development of NEC.[34]

Another ideal use of BUS is for the detection of abdominal ascites because the high-resolution detection of abdominal fluid by US is a well-known superior asset. The ability to detect the presence of clear or particulate fluid is helpful in determining whether a bowel perforation has taken place.[35] Accompanying bowel wall changes, such as thickening and dilatation, greatly increase the suspicion for peritonitis from a perforation.

OTHER MODALITIES

Other modalities have been evaluated to assess bowel in newborns with suspected NEC. These include CT and MRI.[36] Although CT may be able to have a limited value with CT imaging due to the risk of radiation exposure and the extraordinary task of

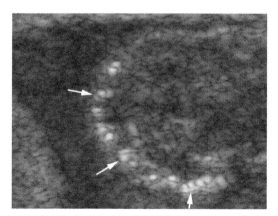

Fig. 2. Pneumatosis intestinalis depicted by BUS. White arrows indicate air bubbles in wall of bowel. (*From* Faingold R, Daneman A, Tomlinson G, et al. Necrotizing enterocolitis: assessment of bowel viability with color doppler US. Radiology 2005;235(2):589; with permission.)

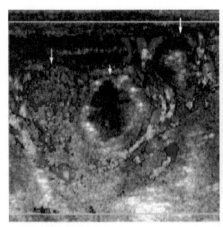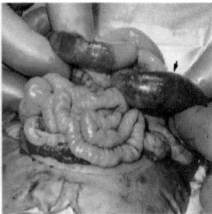

Fig. 3. BUS in NEC. Left panel: white arrows indicate single bowel loops; center white arrow identifies non-perfused necrotic loop of bowel with pneumatosis. Right panel: black arrow shows loop of necrotic bowel at laparotomy. (*From* Epelman M, Daneman A, Navarro OM, et al. Necrotizing enterocolitis: review of state-of-the-art imaging findings with pathologic correlation. Radiographics 2007;27(2):302; with permission.)

moving a sick neonate to a CT scanner, MRI is equally challenging to reach if not close to the unit and for the time it takes to scan. These modalities are not likely to supersede the bedside advantage of US.

ROLE OF RADIOLOGIST AND NEONATOLOGIST/SURGEON

Some surgical or regional neonatal ICUs in North America have started to incorporate BUS into their assessment and management of suspected NEC. This is mostly done by diagnostic imaging where technologists and radiologists are trained to scan and read what NEC may look like on sonogram. The value of BUS performed by a neonatal provider or surgeon is still too early to determine. For NEC, the general availability of US by diagnostic imaging departments means that for most concerns for NEC can be managed by ordering an abdominal US.

SUMMARY

Imaging is a critical component in the diagnosis and management of NEC. The current standard and emphasis on AR, however, are inadequate to meet more accurate aims to assist the diagnosis and optimal surgical management of NEC. Many other imaging modalities have been evaluated, including CT and MRI, but BUS holds great promise over AR and these other modes. BUS for NEC has been described for more than a decade but there has been little traction in implementing BUS as part of routine care for bowel injury, suspected NEC, and NEC. There are enough convincing data currently to start the process of implementing the routine use of BUS during NEC evaluation. What may be required to accelerate the adoption is introducing a structured approach to the implementation of interrogation of bowel in neonates through enhanced training in diagnostic imaging. This may permit a consistent and validated way of recording the various aspects of bowel in health and disease.

Parallel to this is training of other providers, such as neonatologists and surgeons, to be able to interpret the imaging acquired with US bowel assessment as well as obtaining basic skills to be able to image real-time BUS to appreciate the static and dynamic nature of bowel in many clinical situations. This training of all these groups in reading and performing US for bowel assessment will take time. Careful evaluation of the quality of the imaging and interpretation is needed but is likely to improve the promise of BUS in identifying threatened bowel, such as NEC, in vulnerable infants.

REFERENCES

1. Cotten CM, Taylor S, Stoll B, et al. Prolonged duration of initial empirical antibiotic treatment is associated with increased rates of necrotizing enterocolitis and death for extremely low birth weight infants. Pediatrics 2009;123(1):58–66.

2. Allocca M, Fiorino G, Bonifacio C, et al. Comparative accuracy of bowel ultrasound versus magnetic resonance enterography in combination with colonoscopy in assessing Crohn's disease and guiding clinical decision-making. J Crohns Colitis 2018. https://doi.org/10.1093/ecco-jcc/jjy093.

3. Carter D, Eliakim R. Feasibility of bedside bowel ultrasound performed by a gastroenterologist for detection and follow-up of inflammatory bowel disease. Isr Med Assoc J 2017;19(3):139–42.

4. Cavalcoli F, Zilli A, Fraquelli M, et al. Small bowel ultrasound beyond inflammatory bowel disease: an updated review of the recent literature. Ultrasound Med Biol 2017;43(9):1741–52.

5. Strobel D, Goertz RS, Bernatik T. Diagnostics in inflammatory bowel disease: ultrasound. World J Gastroenterol 2011;17(27):3192–7.

6. Sousa HT, Brito J, Magro F. New cross-sectional imaging in IBD. Curr Opin Gastroenterol 2018;34(4):194–207.

7. Rispo A, Imperatore N, Testa A, et al. Diagnostic accuracy of ultrasonography in the detection of postsurgical recurrence in crohn's disease: a systematic review with meta-analysis. Inflamm Bowel Dis 2018;24(5):977–88.

8. Gottlieb M, Peksa GD, Pandurangadu AV, et al. Utilization of ultrasound for the evaluation of small bowel obstruction: a systematic review and meta-analysis. Am J Emerg Med 2018;36(2):234–42.

9. Unluer EE, Yavasi O, Eroglu O, et al. Ultrasonography by emergency medicine and radiology residents for the diagnosis of small bowel obstruction. Eur J Emerg Med 2010;17(5):260–4.

10. Benabbas R, Hanna M, Shah J, et al. Diagnostic accuracy of history, physical examination, laboratory tests, and point-of-care ultrasound for pediatric acute appendicitis in the emergency department: a systematic review and meta-analysis. Acad Emerg Med 2017;24(5):523–51.

11. Koumanidou C, Vakaki M, Pitsoulakis G, et al. Sonographic measurement of the abdominal esophagus length in infancy: a diagnostic tool for gastroesophageal reflux. AJR Am J Roentgenol 2004;183(3):801–7.

12. Pezzati M, Filippi L, Psaraki M, et al. Diagnosis of gastro-oesophageal reflux in preterm infants: sonography vs. pH-monitoring. Neonatology 2007;91(3):162–6.

13. Bozzetti V, Paterlini G, De Lorenzo P, et al. Impact of continuous vs bolus feeding on splanchnic perfusion in very low birth weight infants: a randomized trial. J Pediatr 2016;176:86–92.e2.

14. Robel-Tillig E, Knupfer M, Pulzer F, et al. Blood flow parameters of the superior mesenteric artery as an early predictor of intestinal dysmotility in preterm infants. Pediatr Radiol 2004;34(12):958–62.

15. Thompson A, Silva CT, Gork AS, et al. Intestinal blood flow by Doppler ultrasound: the impact of gestational age and time from first enteral feeding in preterm neonates. Am J Perinatol 2014;31(4):261–8.

16. Zhang W, Sun H, Luo F. The efficiency of sonography in diagnosing volvulus in neonates with suspected intestinal malrotation. Medicine (Baltimore) 2017; 96(42):e8287.

17. Richburg DA, Kim JH. Real-time bowel ultrasound to characterize intestinal motility in the preterm neonate. J Perinatol 2013;33(8):605–8.

18. Hashem RH, Mansi YA, Almasah NS, et al. Doppler ultrasound assessment of the splanchnic circulation in preterms with neonatal sepsis at risk for necrotizing enterocolitis. J Ultrasound 2017;20(1):59–67.

19. Murdoch EM, Sinha AK, Shanmugalingam ST, et al. Doppler flow velocimetry in the superior mesenteric artery on the first day of life in preterm infants and the risk of neonatal necrotizing enterocolitis. Pediatrics 2006;118(5):1999–2003.

20. Urboniene A, Palepsaitis A, Uktveris R, et al. Doppler flowmetry of the superior mesenteric artery and portal vein: impact for the early prediction of necrotizing enterocolitis in neonates. Pediatr Surg Int 2015;31(11):1061–6.

21. Aliev MM, Dekhqonboev AA, Yuldashev RZ. Advantages of abdominal ultrasound in the management of infants with necrotizing enterocolitis. Pediatr Surg Int 2017;33(2):213–6.

22. Cuna AC, Reddy N, Robinson AL, et al. Bowel ultrasound for predicting surgical management of necrotizing enterocolitis: a systematic review and meta-analysis. Pediatr Radiol 2017. https://doi.org/10.1007/s00247-017-4056-x.

23. Dilli D, Suna Oguz S, Erol R, et al. Does abdominal sonography provide additional information over abdominal plain radiography for diagnosis of necrotizing enterocolitis in neonates? Pediatr Surg Int 2011;27(3):321–7.

24. Epelman M, Daneman A, Navarro OM, et al. Necrotizing enterocolitis: review of state-of-the-art imaging findings with pathologic correlation. Radiographics 2007;27(2):285–305.

25. Faingold R, Daneman A, Tomlinson G, et al. Necrotizing enterocolitis: assessment of bowel viability with color Doppler US. Radiology 2005;235(2):587–94.

26. Garbi-Goutel A, Brevaut-Malaty V, Panuel M, et al. Prognostic value of abdominal sonography in necrotizing enterocolitis of premature infants born before 33 weeks gestational age. J Pediatr Surg 2014;49(4):508–13.

27. Kamali K, Hosseini SR, Ardakani SM, et al. Complementory value of sonography in early evaluation of necrotizing enterocolitis. Pol J Radiol 2015;80:317–23.

28. Muchantef K, Epelman M, Darge K, et al. Sonographic and radiographic imaging features of the neonate with necrotizing enterocolitis: correlating findings with outcomes. Pediatr Radiol 2013. https://doi.org/10.1007/s00247-013-2725-y.

29. Silva CT, Daneman A, Navarro OM, et al. Correlation of sonographic findings and outcome in necrotizing enterocolitis. Pediatr Radiol 2007;37(3):274–82.

30. Staryszak J, Stopa J, Kucharska-Miasik I, et al. Usefulness of ultrasound examinations in the diagnostics of necrotizing enterocolitis. Pol J Radiol 2015;80:1–9.

31. Wang L, Li Y, Liu J. Diagnostic value and disease evaluation significance of abdominal ultrasound inspection for neonatal necrotizing enterocolitis. Pak J Med Sci 2016;32(5):1251–6.

32. Yang L, Xu W, Li YW, et al. Value of abdominal ultrasound in the diagnosis of neonatal necrotizing enterocolitis and evaluation of disease severity. Zhongguo Dang Dai Er Ke Za Zhi 2016;18(2):108–12 [in Chinese].

33. Bohnhorst B, Kuebler JF, Rau G, et al. Portal venous gas detected by ultrasound differentiates surgical NEC from other acquired neonatal intestinal diseases. Eur J Pediatr Surg 2011;21(1):12–7.
34. Chen S, Hu Y, Liu Q, et al. Comparison of abdominal radiographs and sonography in prognostic prediction of infants with necrotizing enterocolitis. Pediatr Surg Int 2018;34(5):535–41.
35. Palleri E, Aghamn I, Bexelius TS, et al. The effect of gestational age on clinical and radiological presentation of necrotizing enterocolitis. J Pediatr Surg 2017. https://doi.org/10.1016/j.jpedsurg.2017.09.018.
36. Maalouf EF, Fagbemi A, Duggan PJ, et al. Magnetic resonance imaging of intestinal necrosis in preterm infants. Pediatrics 2000;105(3 Pt 1):510–4.

Modifiable Risk Factors in Necrotizing Enterocolitis

C. Michael Cotten, MD, MHS

KEYWORDS

- Necrotizing enterocolitis • Breastfeeding • Human milk • Quality improvement
- Antibiotics • Antacids • Transfusions

KEY POINTS

- Neonatologists and neonatal ICU (NICU) caregivers can modify practices and develop consistent approaches to clinical problems based on clinical trial and cohort studies and knowledge of physiology and, by doing so, can improve outcomes.
- Cooperative, informed, well-planned, unified efforts of neonatologists and all others providing care for premature infants can often modify and optimize practice and identify and overcome obstacles to improve outcomes.
- Optimizing provision of mother's milk feeding of premature infants via multiple mechanisms and approaches is likely to result in reductions in rates of necrotizing enterocolitis in NICUs where mother's own breast milk feeding of preterm infants' rates are low.
- Multiple other aspects of care, including transfusion-related practices and medication uses and feeding protocol, likely will be influenced by ongoing and recently completed clinical trials.
- Dissemination of results and understanding site practices and outcomes relative to others will be key in identifying next meaningful steps toward reduction in NEC among preterm infants.

INTRODUCTION: DEFINING NECROTIZING ENTEROCOLITIS

For this review, NEC is considered as medical NEC and surgical NEC. On a deeper level, NEC is considered a spectrum of disease manifested by injury of the intestinal mucosa, invasion of the intestinal tissue by microbes with a substantial inflammatory response, pneumatosis intestinalis, and coagulative necrosis of the mucosa with focal hemorrhage (medical NEC). The most extreme cases include rupture of necrotic intestine and release of intestinal contents into the peritoneum (surgical NEC).[1] This overall NEC phenotype has classically been summarized as NEC class IIA or higher,

Disclosure Statement: The author received support from the Eunice Kennedy Shriver NICHD, grant # 5UG1-HD040492-18, for the Neonatal Research Network.
Department of Pediatrics, Division of Neonatal-Perinatal Medicine, Duke University School of Medicine, Box 2739 DUMC, Durham, NC 27710, USA
E-mail address: Michael.cotten@duke.edu

Clin Perinatol 46 (2019) 129–143
https://doi.org/10.1016/j.clp.2018.10.007
0095-5108/19/© 2018 Elsevier Inc. All rights reserved.

consistent with modified Bell's staging criteria, the criteria used in multicenter reports summarizing NEC rates globally for decades.[2–5] Although ultrasound has promising preliminary evidence supporting its utility for diagnosis of medical NEC,[6,7] a diagnosis of medical NEC in this review is based primarily on the presence of pneumatosis intestinalis or hepatobiliary air on plain films, acknowledging that these carry some degree of reader variability.[8–10] Some investigators have suggested modifying the taxonomy regarding acquired neonatal intestinal diseases, which more strictly separates surgical NEC from spontaneous perforation.[11,12] This classification acknowledges that surgical NEC usually includes gross and microscopic evidence of pneumatosis or tissue necrosis and does not include isolated intestinal perforations.

THE NECROTIZING ENTEROCOLITIS RATE IS CHANGING

Recent large cohort studies of extremely preterm infants, by the US Eunice Kennedy Shriver National Institute of Child Health and Human Development (NICHD) Neonatal Research Network (NRN), the Pediatrix Medical Group, the Vermont Oxford Network (Burlington, Vermont) (VON), and the Canadian Neonatal Network (CNN) indicate a mostly positive picture of decreasing NEC rates (data summarized in **Table 1**).[5,13–16] In the recent summary of NRN data inclusive of infants 22 weeks' to 28 weeks' gestation born at NRN sites and who survived beyond the first 12 postnatal hours, the medical plus surgical NEC rates were 11% from 1993 - 1997, 9% from 1998 - 2002, 9% from 2203 - 2007, and 10% from 2008 – 2012. More specific single-year data included in the NRN report suggest improvement within that time period, with a NEC rate 13% (187 of 1496) in 2008 and 9% (161 of 1756) by 2012.[5] The VON, incorporating 408,164 very-low-birth-weight infants (VLBW) (<1500-g birthweight) from 756 hospitals in its data set, reported that 76% of the hospitals achieved shrunken adjusted rates of medical NEC plus surgical NEC as low as or lower than the rate of the best-performing quartile of hospitals in 2005.[14] VON has provided more granular data, reporting the rate of medical NEC plus surgical NEC for all infants included in the VON database who were born at VON centers from 2007 to 2017. The rate seems to be decreasing among all the infants less than 1500-g birthweight, including both the extremely low birthweight infants (ELBW; <1000 g birthweight) and those born weighing 1000 g to 1500 g (VON Very Low Birthweight Database, unpublished data, 2018; used with permission).

WHICH RISK FACTORS?

Three factors are generally regarded as necessarily present for NEC: (1) an immature bowel colonized with microorganisms, (2) food in the bowel, and (3) a trigger event that compromises the integrity of the mucosal barrier.[1] Additional risk factors, not controllable by neonatologists, include gestational age, birth weight, and possibly genetic variation.[17–19] That said multiple decisions are made during the NICU stay of preterm infants. Choices made, particularly around feeding and medication use and the environment neonatal intensive caregivers and institutions provide, influence the 3 NEC factors, and many of these choices have been targets of interventions by various multicenter groups as well as single-center efforts.[4,13,20–24] The practice modifications include aspects of feeding strategies (when feedings are initiated and how fast they are increased), controlling use of antibiotics, and controlling use of antacids. In addition to practice modifications and considerations, such as when to start feedings or stop an empirical antibiotic course, enlisting and optimizing universal, comprehensive individual and institutional support, which facilitates a mother's ability to provide milk for her baby, has been an integral modification of neonatologists' daily practice and an

Table 1
Necrotizing enterocolitis (medical plus surgical) rates in multicenter consortia, 1993–2017

Data Source Cohort characteristic	Data Source Years														
	1993–1997	1998–2002	2003–2007	2008–2012	2007	2008	2009	2010	2011	2012	2013	2014	2015	2016	2017
NICHD[5]															
ELBW, <29 wk inborn	9%	9%	11%	10%											
Overall NRN rate															
CNN[4,15] *(2 reports)*	*1996–1997*		*2006–2007*												
<29 wk	7.5%		7.0%					9.6%	9.1%	8.6%	7.6%				
Pediatrix[13]					*2007*	*2008*	*2009*	*2010*	*2011*	*2012*	*2013*				
501–1500 g					6.6%	6.4%	5.4%	5.5%	4.9%	4%	3.9%				
VON[14]					*2007*	*2008*	*2009*	*2010*	*2011*	*2012*	*2013*				
VLBW inborn + outborn					7.2%[a]	7[a]	6.5[a]	6.2[a]	5.9[a]	5.7[a]	5[a]				
VON Very Low Birthweight Database, unpublished data, 2018; used with permission					*2007*	*2008*	*2009*	*2010*	*2011*	*2012*	*2013*	*2014*	*2015*	*2016*	*2017*
All VLBW inborns					6.8%	6.6%	5.9%	5.8%	5.2%	4.8%	4.3%	4.5%	4.2%	4.1%	4.0%
ELBW (<1000 grams BW only)					10.4%	10.7%	9.4%	9.2%	8.2%	7.8%	6.9%	7.3%	6.8%	7.0%	6.6%
1000–1500 grams birthweight only					4.1%	3.8%	3.4%	3.3%	3.1%	2.7%	2.6%	2.5%	2.3%	2.0%	2.2%

[a] Mean rate per center.

advocacy priority.[25] Finally, activities and intervention decisions with varying degrees of certainty of their contributions to NEC risk, such as transfusion practice, feeding around transfusions, and use of probiotics, have been included in bundles of care targeting reduction in NEC, with varying degrees of success.[17]

SUCCESS STORIES RELATED TO MODIFYING PRACTICES: MULTISITE STUDIES
Ohio Collaborative

From 2010 to 2013, a group of 8 affiliated hospitals in the state of Ohio set out to use quality-improvement (QI) methodologies to reduce NEC from their baseline of 8% among VLBW infants. They targeted 3 areas for practice modification: (1) standardize early human milk feedings, (2) implement conservative feeding guidelines during blood transfusions and indomethacin treatment, and (3) restrict ranitidine use in VLBW infants. The percentage of infants fed their own mother's milk on or before postnatal day 3 increased from 0% before September 2010, to 30% by October 2010–September 2011, and to 50% by January 2012. For transfusions, the report[20] does not provide transfusion guidelines but states that feeds were held during transfusions, and neither volume nor fortification was advanced the same day as a transfusion. Participating sites also limited feeds during indomethacin treatment of patent ductus arteriosus. The investigators did not provide quantitative results of emphasizing the restricted ranitidine use policy; however, the investigators stated that "compliance with this policy before the QI initiative was poor. During the QI initiative, compliance with restricted ranitidine use in VLBW infants improved." These hospitals started with an overall baseline rate of NEC of 8% (27 NEC cases among 335 VLBW infants). After implementation of the QI efforts, NEC prevalence was 3.1% (19 of 606 VLBW infants) from November 2011 to December 2013. NEC-related mortality decreased from 2.7% to 0.9%.[20]

California Perinatal Quality Care Collaborative

Eleven sites in the California Perinatal Quality Care Collaborative (CPQCC) took on the challenge to improve breastfeeding rates, by implementing self-selected interventions, with the secondary aim of reducing NEC. They compared baseline (October 2008–September 2009), implementation (October 2009–September 2010), and sustainability (October 2010–March 2011) periods' rates of breastfeeding success (breastfeeding at discharge) and NEC rates in the same eras. The study population included infants 401 g to 1500 g at birth, or 22 weeks' to 29 weeks' gestational age, admitted between October 1, 2008, and March 31, 2011, either inborn or outborn, and transferred into a CPQCC NICU within 48 hours of birth. At participating sites, the overall rate of discharge on breastmilk improved from baseline (54.6%, SD 49.8%) to the sustainability phase (64.0%, SD 48.1%; $P = .003$). Practices that were adopted at all participating hospitals that had been in place in fewer than 50% of these sites prior to the project included (1) daily recommendations of skin-to-skin contact; (2) breastmilk feeding information was provided to all mothers, and (3) advice given to mothers on manual expression. Eight hospitals instituted oral colostrum protocols. Nine hospitals increased breast milk feeding rates during the intervention and sustainability periods combined, whereas 2 hospitals decreased. Mean NEC rates decreased during the implementation phase (7.0% to 4.3%; $P = .02$), with continued decrease during the sustainability phase (2.4%; $P<.0001$). Compared with baseline, 8 hospitals had decreased NEC rates in the intervention and sustainability periods combined, 2 hospitals increased, and 1 hospital remained the same. In multivariable analyses adjusting for sociodemographic and medical risk factors, there was a 44%

increase in odds of breast milk feeding at discharge and 74% decrease in odds of NEC for participants during the sustainability phase compared with baseline.[21]

Canadian Neonatal Network

Between 2008 and 2012, 25 NICUs in the CNN conducted a prospective cohort study implementing use of the Evidence-based Practice for Improving Quality (EPIQ) approach to care.[4] The investigators summarize this approach as combining use of the best available evidence with institution-specific data to identify institution-specific needs. This project was an expansion of the EPIQ approach taken in earlier successful work at 12 CNN hospitals, which demonstrated reduction nosocomial infections and bronchopulmonary dysplasia.[26] For the 2008 to 2012 study, the primary outcome was a composite of death or any of 5 major morbidities. NEC stage II or greater was one of the targeted morbidities.[2,4] Training in QI methodologies was provided across all disciplines of NICU care teams, and feedback was provided every few months on baseline data, selected outcomes over time, and process and intervention success rates. As information was provided, interventions would be adapted. Sites choose multiple interventions that were classified based on level of supportive evidence: definitive, nondefinitive, and unsubstantiated. Among the 130 practice changes targeting a specific outcome and 30 interventions aimed at improved care process, several targeted NEC. Eleven sites developed feeding guidelines. Other aspects adopted at 1 to 6 sites included early feeding, use of donor milk, use of colostrum or enhancing expressed milk, early use of total parenteral nutrition, and holding feeds during transfusions. Other interventions targeting other outcomes and implemented by 10 or more sites included using central line care bundles, improving hand hygiene, and controlling oxygen use. Comparing the third year of the project with the baseline year, the composite outcome was reduced by year 3. In multivariable analysis, NEC was reduced (OR 0.73; 95%, CI 0.52–0.98 and NNT 50; 95% CI, 25–714). The majority of improvement was noted in infants born at 26 weeks' to 28 weeks' gestational age. At the sites implementing enhanced use of colostrum or enhanced expressed breast milk feeding, NEC risk decreased 5.3% (95% CI, 1.9–8.9). Details of the modifications to colostrum protocols and methods to enhance expressed milk use are not included in the article.[4]

Pediatrix Medical Group

In the largest of the QI projects, the Pediatrix Medical Group, a private practice group of physicians providing neonatal intensive care in diverse types of nurseries in 34 US states and in Puerto Rico, set out to modify care to reduce mortality and morbidities associated with extreme prematurity. Methodologies included providing transparency for sites to examine their own data as well as overall Pediatrix network data, to track outcomes. Sites chose among multiple projects and approaches. Pediatrix provided quality summits 3 times per year, with invited experts in pathophysiology of the problems associated with extreme prematurity, the epidemiology, and current clinical research regarding major morbidities of prematurity as well as methodologies specific for QI science. Over the 6 years of the study period (2007–2013), Pediatrix provided care to 58,555 infants with birthweight between 500 g and 1500 g. Their achieved goals of care included increasing prevalence of any human milk feeding (donor or maternal milk) from 77% in 2007 to 88% in 2013 and increased prevalence of use of human milk at discharge from 42% in 2007 to 53% in 2013. The group also successfully reduced exposures to several medications, including H_2-blockers (from 17% in 2007–7% in 2013) metoclopramide (from 20.8% in 2007–1.1% in 2013). They decreased rates of preterm infants with sterile initial blood cultures continuing antibiotics beyond the third postnatal day from 35% in 2007 to 28% in 2013. The proportion of infants treated with mechanical ventilation and the number of days of ventilator support for those mechanically ventilated both decreased. Over the intervention period, NEC decreased from 6.6% in 2007 to 3.9% in 2013. Surgical NEC decreased from 2.2% in 2007 to 1.2% in 2013. Mortality, surgical retinopathy of prematurity (ROP), and bacteremia after postnatal day 3 all decreased, and survival without significant morbidity (NEC, severe intraventricular hemorrhage, severe ROP, and oxygen use at 36 weeks) improved. Weight gain improved, and length of hospital stay among discharge was increased.[13]

There is some consistency of increasing human milk feeding, reducing exposures to certain medications, and frequently a reduction in infection that corresponds with the reduction in NEC rates. Targets for practice change and the noted changes in practice and changes in NEC and in other noted outcomes are summarized in **Table 2**.

SINGLE-SITE STUDIES: NOT ALWAYS IMMEDIATELY SUCCESSFUL

In a presentation to the VON Internet-based Newborn Improvement Collaborative for Quality (iNICQ), monthly webinar in the antibiotic stewardship series in 2018, Dr Ravi Patel described a single-site QI project that aimed to reduce NEC from 15% to 5% among VLBW infants from 2013 to 2018. Targeted interventions included delayed cord clamping, adherence to a revised feeding protocol, increasing maternal breastfeeding, using donor milk in the absence of mother's milk, and reducing antacid use and decreasing prolonged antibiotic use. They also incorporated use of a probiotic, *Lactobacillus rhamnosus* GG (ATCC 53103) (LGG) at doses consistent with clinical trials.[23,27,28] Acid suppression use (the first targeted process) decreased from 27% to 0%, delayed cord clamping increased from 0% to 82%, and probiotic use was initiated in 2013, with 88% exposure. Exposure to any human milk improved from 89% to 100% and donor milk exposure increased from 0% to 28%. Before 2017, 41% of VLBW infants were on antibiotics beyond their first 48 postnatal hours, and, afterward, the percentage was 29%. Over time, inclusive of implementation of the practice changes, from 2008 to 2018, the mean rate of NEC remained 13%.[28] The investigators of the published report hypothesized that the unchanging/increasing NEC could be related to unmeasured differences in patient characteristics or clinical practice over time that were associated with both LGG supplementation and NEC. They conclude that their findings highlight the need for additional studies to evaluate probiotic products, product quality, timing of initiation, and interactions with human milk feeding and antibiotic use to better understand the treatment effects of probiotics on NEC.[23]

In another example, in 2009 the clinical team at Rush University instituted a QI initiative to reduce NEC among VLBW infants from their 4% baseline rate. Rush University has maintained a highly successful rate of mother's milk feeding.[29] Their plan included an evidence-based feeding protocol; however, in the intervention phase, the rate of medical NEC plus surgical NEC increased to 10%. On examination, the QI teams identified a change in feeding tube practice, with initiation of use of feeding tubes that remained in place for up to 30 days. In addition, initiation of feedings in the first 3 postnatal days decreased from 43% in the baseline period to 18% in the first QI epoch when NEC increased. In reviewing the literature, the team at Rush noted evidence for association between nasogastric tube dwell time and colonization of the tube with gram-negative rods and subsequently with NEC.[30,31] A second set of QI initiatives based on findings of examinations of care practices followed, with an emphasis on maximizing support to obtain early feedings with colostrum and a change in feeding tube practice to weekly tube changes instead of 30 days. In this second QI phase,

Table 2
Targeted risk factors for multicenter quality-improvement projects resulting in decreased necrotizing enterocolitis

Quality-Improvement Report	Project Characteristics	Practice Changes	Outcome Changes
Talavera et al,[20] 2016	2010–2012 VLBW infants 8 sites; n = 941	1. Standardized early human milk feedings 2. Conservative feeding guidelines during blood transfusions and indomethacin treatment 3. Restricted ranitidine use in VLBW infants	Decreased NEC and NEC-related mortality
Lee et al,[21] 2012	2008–2011 VLBW infants 11 intervention sites 88 control sites; n = unknown	1. Daily recommendations of skin-to-skin contact 2. Breastmilk feeding information provided to all mothers 3. Advice on manual express 4. Hospital policies to support breast milk feeding 5. Early use/mouth care with expressed milk 6. Begin trophic feeds early (hours to days) 7. Monitored milk supplies	Increased odds of breast milk feeding at discharge Decreased NEC (7.4% to 2.4%) Length of stay, increased
Lee et al,[4] 2014	2008–2012 <29-wk gestational age 25 NICUs; n = 6026	EPIQ interventions inclusive of 1. Establishing feeding guidelines 2. Central line bundles 3. Hand hygiene 4. Controlled oxygen use	Lowered NEC Lowered composite outcome: death or NEC, BPD, severe neurologic injury, severe ROP, or nosocomial infection
Ellsbury et al,[13] 2016	2007–2013 501–1500 g birthweight 300 + NICUs; n = 58,555	Bolstered QI culture Five targets 1. More breastfeeding through discharge 2. Shorter duration of antibiotics with sterile cultures 3. Fewer medications (dexamethasone, antacids, metoclopramide, and cefotaxime) 4. Minimize ventilator exposure 5. Feeding protocols, early protein in IV 6. Central line insertion and maintenance bundles 7. Improve thermal management at delivery	Decreased Mortality NEC ROP Bacteremia after postnatal day 3 CLABSI Improved Survival without significant morbidity (NEC, severe ROP, severe IVH, oxygen use at 36 wk), decreased

Abbreviations: BPD: Bronchopulmonary dysplasia; CLABSI: Central line-associated bloodstream infection; IVH: intraventricular hemorrhage.

prevalence of feedings within the first 3 postnatal days increased to 49%, and, along with the change in feeding tube practice changes, the rate of surgical NEC cases progressively declined from 5% in the baseline phase to 4.8% in QI phase 1 and to 1.2% in QI phase 2. During the baseline period, the prevalence of late-onset sepsis unrelated to NEC among the VLBW cohort was 11%. During the first QI phase, with the long feeding tube dwell times, the prevalence of late-onset sepsis was 24%, and, during the last period, late-onset sepsis decreased to 9%. This report is remarkable, because it demonstrates the importance of assessing multiple factors and aspects of care to identify what might be contributing to risk, modifying that practice, and then assessing and reporting the changes in practice, the change in the target outcome, and the changes in balancing measures. For those aiming for successful initiation and support of mothers providing their own milk, at least early in the NICU study, more than 97% of infants received any mother's milk feeding throughout the baseline, first QI, and second QI epochs.[22]

WHAT IS KNOWN ABOUT MODIFICATION OF RISK FACTORS AND WHICH TO PRIORITIZE?

In 2010, Christensen and colleagues[32] speculated that 2 prevention strategies shown in meta-analyses or observational cohort studies to reduce the incidence of NEC were not being fully used. One was to implement programs to increase the availability of human milk for patients at risk of developing NEC. The second was implementing a written set of feeding guidelines (also called standardized feeding regimens) for NICU patients.[32–34] Consistent with these speculations, Rose and Patel[17] recently published a review of more than 40 risk factors for NEC, including maternal characteristics, antenatal exposures, infant characteristics (demographic, birthweight, and gestational age), delivery room events, postnatal clinical events and exposures, and feeding approaches and exposures. As cited in their report, a recent survey of dozens of experts arrived at agreement on only 3 consensus risk factors for NEC. Little can be done by neonatologists about the first 2 risk factors, birthweight and gestational age, all NICU caregivers can contribute to efforts to maximize use of mothers milk over formula.[35]

Improving Use of Mother's Own Milk in the Neonatal Intensive Care Unit

On a broad scale in the QI reports, improvement in sustained provision of human milk was associated with decreasing NEC rates. The QI efforts summarized in this review all included approaches emphasizing use of human milk for feeding. The CPQCC initiative in particular is notable for its success in improving mothers' ability to provide milk to their babies. Approximately 50% of infants breastfeeding at discharge at the beginning of the project. At the finish, approximately two-thirds of babies were discharged home receiving human milk. Their projects incorporated 22 practices and activities geared toward optimizing breastfeeding rates. They included efforts to educate/advocate for human milk for (all) NICU infants and comprehensive efforts for staff and administration to support mothers in establishing and maintaining maternal milk supplies. The details include approaches to educate parents about the importance of breastmilk, enhance and support collection and storage, and support bedside pumping.[21] These all require significant commitment, from every individual working with families and in the NICU space, including up to the highest administrative levels, where decisions regarding allotments of space, resources, and personnel are made. These investments are likely to be justified by cost savings among NICU infants fed more human milk than formula, even from a hospital perspective.[36–38]

In a recent systematic review of implementation strategies to reduce NEC, Gephart and colleagues[39] used the translating research into practice framework to assess modifiable practices for levels of evidence. Their results indicated that prioritizing human milk and using feeding protocols as well as avoiding antacids were strongly recommended. Weaker recommendations were made to develop and implement strategies to limit antibiotic use and to develop and implement timely NEC recognition strategies. Although changing direction of decisions regarding use of medications is relatively straightforward, Gephart and colleagues' review is a reminder that working to optimize mothers providing milk is much more complex. Although it may be challenging, providing milk has the strongest consensus of what to optimize to minimize NEC risk. In their review, 14 specific interventions are discussed, some similar to those listed in the CPQCC QI report. They also include suggestions that require multidisciplinary support and participation, such as for staff to support initiation of pumping within 6 hours after delivery and to offer pumping at the bedside when possible. Also they recommend institutions provide lactation specialist support early (first 24 postnatal hours) and consistently through the stay, prioritize staff education (inclusive of nursing, medical, and administrative staff) using diverse training tools, and provide pumps in the hospital and resources for mothers to rent pumps at home.[21,39] An extremely comprehensive review of the QI approaches to improving rates of mothers successfully providing their own milk to their infants in the NICU was recently published.[40] The most recent Cochrane analysis on feeding donor milk versus preterm formula to preterm infants concluded that feeding with formula compared with donor breast milk, either as a supplement to maternal expressed breast milk or as a sole diet, results in increased rates of NEC but also higher rates of weight gain, linear growth, and head growth, with no known impact on neurodevelopmental outcome.[41]

In addition to optimizing feeding with human milk, standardizing feeding protocols among providers has been associated with reductions in NEC risk over several decades, and the spread of making feedings within institutions consistent may be contributing to the trend toward reduction in rates of NEC.[33,42,43] In deciding what the feeding practices should be, starting feeds in the first postnatal days seems to improve intestinal adaptation to extrauterine life in animal models and in human infants.[44–46] Although this background indicates early feeding is important, the most recent Cochrane analysis of early (first 4 postnatal days) versus later initiation of enteral feeds did not identify a clear advantage; however, the investigators acknowledge a paucity of the most preterm infants, at highest risk of NEC in the studies included in the analysis.[47] In another single-site QI study focused on supporting breastfeeding and provide early postnatal supplemental donor human milk and probiotics to preterm infants, NEC was decreased, and the association its association with prolonged antibiotic exposure was blunted.[24]

Modifying Medication Exposures

Medication exposures, in particular use of antibiotics and ranitidine use, were targeted for reduction in the Ohio group and the Pediatrix Medical Group reports as well as Patel's single-center report.[13,20,23,28] Antibiotics are the most commonly used class of medications used in the intensive care nursery, particularly for extremely preterm infants. Virtually all are exposed at some point in their NICU stay, particularly in the first postnatal days.[48] Antibiotic duration, in the setting of sterile initial cultures, has been associated with higher risk of NEC in multiple retrospective cohort studies, as summarized in a recent systematic review.[49] One potential mechanism is that antibiotics influence the diversity of the intestinal microbiome, and contribute to the development of resistant species of microbiota.[50] Among the reviewed reports, antibiotic use was decreased in the Pediatrix medical group's cohort, and NEC, late-onset sepsis, and mortality all decreased.[13] Several groups have reported reductions in duration of the initial antibiotic course for preterm infants since publication of the studies identifying associations between longer antibiotic courses in the setting of sterile initial cultures.[51–53] A recent notable single center QI effort from the United Kingdom reduced the antibiotic use rate by 43%, and the proportion of culture-negative sepsis screens where antibiotics were stopped within 36 hours to 48 hours increased consistently from a baseline of 32.5% to 91%. For the period of the QI project implementation, among the VLBW infants, mortality rate and NEC rate were the lowest the site had ever recorded.[54] Recent analysis of the NICHD NRN cohort of infants of birthweight less than 1000-g birthweight and less than 29 weeks' gestation who survived beyond 12 postnatal hours found that early-onset sepsis prevalence was 29 of 5640 (0.5%) among low-risk infants, defined as those delivered via cesarean delivery, with membrane rupture at delivery, and with absence of clinical chorioamnionitis. The remainder of the cohort had a much higher prevalence of early-onset sepsis (209 of 8422 [2.5%]; adjusted relative risk = 0.24 [95% CI, 0.16–0.36]).[55] This low-risk group could be a target for further efforts to study modification of antibiotic use.

Antacid exposure has decreased considerably in reports of medication use in NICUs. The exposure rate to ranitidine in the Pediatrix Medical Group NICU ELBW infants was 293 infants per 1000 in 2005 and decreased to 141 per 1000 ELBW infants in 2010.[48] Patel reported decrease in ranitidine use, as did the multisite report from Pediatrix Medical Group.[13,22] Retrospective cohort studies had suggested an association between NEC and prior exposure to antacids.[56,57] Data on its efficacy to improve cardiorespiratory problems believed attributable to gastroesophageal reflux have not been compelling in 1 double-blind randomized trial of metoclopramide plus ranitidine versus placebo; infants receiving the medications demonstrated more cardiorespiratory instability than those receiving placebo.[58]

Transfusion Practices

Transfusion among extremely preterm infants and their association with NEC is a hot topic among neonatologists, with evidence from cohort studies suggesting associations between transfusions and NEC in the days after transfusion and a meta-analysis of clinical trials of maintaining high versus low transfusion thresholds not showing a strong impact of more versus fewer transfusions used to maintain goal hematocrit in clinical trials.[59–62] Among the cohort studies, in 1 study of 600 VLBW infants, there was a strong association between having severe anemia (hemoglobin <8 mg/dL) in a given week in the NICU and subsequent NEC.[63] Several reports identify transfusions in the settings of extreme anemia as adding more risk than transfusions at higher hematocrits[64,65]; however, a recent cohort study has been added to others that did not find associations between feeding fortification volume increase or packed red blood cells transfusion within 48 hours prior to NEC onset and onset of NEC.[66–68]

Although associations between transfusions and NEC have been the subject of the debate, the associations between feeding during transfusions and NEC have also been a hot topic.[62,69] The Ohio collaborative project included holding feeds during transfusion.[20] In a report of 1380 VLBW infants admitted to a single tertiary NICU, DeRienzo and colleagues[65] noted a decrease in NEC after initiation of a hold feeds during transfusion policy (126/939[12%] to 22/293 [7%]; $P = .01$), but on further scrutiny, the percentage of NEC cases occurring within 48 hours of transfusion in the pre-policy and postpolicy implementation periods was not significantly different (51/126 [41%] versus 9/22 [41%], P>.99). Identifying the optimal threshold for transfusion and whether or not to feed during transfusion are decisions clinicians are making in

NICUs daily. For the optimal hemoglobin/hematocrit at which to transfuse, a multi-center study Transfusions of Prematures (TOP), which enrolled more than 1800 ELBW infants, has completed enrollment and is in its follow-up phase (https://clinicaltrials.gov/ct2/show/NCT01702805). The definitive, gold standard evidence to support holding enteral feeds during transfusions will have to wait for the definitive trial. The TOP trial may also provide useful information regarding the impact of holding feeds during PRBC transfusions on risk of NEC.[70]

SUMMARY

Evidence supporting the ability of neonatologists and their NICU colleagues to mean-ingfully change practice and improve mothers' ability to provide their own milk to their own babies, to cooperate and follow feeding protocols consistently, and to alter their use of medications is convincing. As the neonatology community, inclusive of all who care for these infants, including parents, work together on particular causes, out-comes are improving. These multicenter efforts translate down to single-center ef-forts, where practice and attitudes change on a 1-by-1 individual basis. Evidence, such as in the NICHD NRN and VON, still clearly demonstrate center variations in prac-tices and outcomes, but they show that some aspects, like breast milk use and medi-cation use, are changing in many NICUs.[5,13,14] With reduction in NEC a common goal, the NICU caregiver community must continue to keep an eye on outcomes of patients and families, be aware of practices and their impact, work to identify best practices, and modify efforts in response to accumulating accurate data on actual practice and outcomes.

REFERENCES

1. Gordon P, Christensen R, Weitkamp JH, et al. Mapping the new world of necro-tizing enterocolitis (NEC): review and opinion. EJ Neonatol Res 2012;2:145–72.
2. Bell MJ, Ternberg JL, Feigin RD, et al. Neonatal necrotizing enterocolitis: thera-peutic decisions based upon clinical staging. Ann Surg 1978;187:1–7.
3. Walsh MC, Kliegman RM. Necrotizing enterocolitis: treatment based on staging criteria. Pediatr Clin North Am 1986;33:179–201.
4. Lee SK, Shah PS, Singhal N, et al, Canadian EPIQ Study Group. Association of a quality improvement program with neonatal outcomes in extremely preterm in-fants: a prospective cohort study. CMAJ 2014;186:E485–94.
5. Stoll BJ, Hansen NI, Bell EF, et al. Trends in care practices, morbidity, and mor-tality of extremely preterm neonates, 1993-2012. JAMA 2015;314:1039–51.
6. Bohnhorst B. Usefulness of abdominal ultrasound in diagnosing necrotising enterocolitis. Arch Dis Child Fetal Neonatal Ed 2013;98(5):F445–50.
7. Ahle M, Ringertz HG, Rubesova E. The role of imaging in the management of ne-crotising enterocolitis: a multispecialist survey and a review of the literature. Eur Radiol 2018;28:3621–31.
8. Rehan VK, Seshia MM, Johnston B, et al. Observer variability in interpretation of abdominal radiographs of infants with suspected necrotizing enterocolitis. Clin Pediatr 1999;38:637–43.
9. Coursey CA, Hollingsworth CL, Gaca AM, et al. Radiologists' agreement when using a 10-point scale to report abdominal radiographic findings of necrotizing enterocolitis in neonates and infants. AJR Am J Roentgenol 2008;191:190–7.
10. Markiet K, Szymanska-Dubowik A, Janczewska I, et al. Agreement and reprodu-cibility of radiological signs in NEC using the duke abdominal assessment scale (DAAS). Pediatr Surg Int 2017;33:335–40.

11. Gordon PV. Understanding intestinal vulnerability to perforation in the extremely low birth weight infant. Pediatr Res 2009;65:138–44.

12. Gordon PV, Swanson JR, Attridge JT, et al. Emerging trends in acquired neonatal intestinal disease: is it time to abandon Bell's criteria? J Perinatol 2007;27:661–71.

13. Ellsbury DL, Clark RH, Ursprung R, et al. A multifaceted approach to improving outcomes in the NICU: the Pediatrix 100000 babies campaign. Pediatrics 2016;137 [pii:e20150389].

14. Horbar JD, Edwards EM, Greenberg LT, et al. Variation in performance of neonatal intensive care units in the United States. JAMA Pediatr 2017;171: e164396.

15. Shah PS, Sankaran K, Aziz K, et al. Outcomes of preterm infants <29 weeks gestation over 10-year period in Canada: a cause for concern? J Perinatol 2012;32:132–8.

16. Battersby C, Santhalingam T, Costeloe K, et al. Incidence of neonatal necrotizing enterocolitis in high-income countries: a systematic review. Arch Dis Child Fetal Neonatal Ed 2018;103:F182–9.

17. Rose AT, Patel RM. A critical analysis of risk factors for necrotizing enterocolitis. Semin Fetal Neonatal Med 2018. https://doi.org/10.1016/j.siny.2018.07.005.

18. Bhandari V, Bizzarro MJ, Shetty A, et al. Familial and genetic susceptibility to major neonatal morbidities in preterm twins. Pediatrics 2006;117:1901–6.

19. Jilling T, Ambalavanan N, Cotten CM, et al. Surgical necrotizing enterocolitis in extremely premature neonates is associated with genetic variations in an intergenic region of chromosome 8. Pediatr Res 2018;83:943–53.

20. Talavera MM, Bixler G, Cozzi C, et al. Quality improvement initiative to reduce the necrotizing enterocolitis rate in premature infants. Pediatrics 2016;137(5): e20151119.

21. Lee HC, Kurtin PS, Wight NE, et al. A quality improvement project to increase breast milk use in very low birth weight infants. Pediatrics 2012. https://doi.org/ 10.1542/peds.2012-0547.

22. Patel AL, Trivedi S, Bhandari NP, et al. Reducing necrotizing enterocolitis in very low birth weight infants using quality-improvement methods. J Perinatol 2014;34: 850–7.

23. Kane AF, Bhatia AD, Denning PW, et al. Routine supplementation of Lactobacillus rhamnosus GG and risk of necrotizing enterocolitis in very low birth weight infants. J Pediatr 2018;195:73–9.

24. Feinberg M, Miller L, Engers B, et al. Reduced necrotizing enterocolitis after an initiative to Promote breastfeeding and early human milk administration. Pediatr Qual Saf 2017;2:e014.

25. Meier PP. Breastfeeding in the special care nursery. Prematures and infants with medical problems. Pediatr Clin North Am 2001;48:425–42.

26. Lee SK, Aziz K, Singhal N, et al. Improving the quality of care for infants: a cluster randomized controlled trial. CMAJ 2009;181:469–76.

27. Patel RM, Denning PW. Therapeutic use of prebiotics, probiotics, and postbiotics to prevent necrotizing enterocolitis: what is the current evidence? Clin Perinatol 2013;40:11–25.

28. Patel R. Available at: https://necsociety.org/2018/07/27/how-to-explain-when-nec-rates-persist-even-when-a-nicu-does-everything-right/. Accessed November 19, 2018.

29. Meier PP, Engstrom JL, Patel AL, et al. Improving the use of human milk during and after the NICU stay. Clin Perinatol 2010;37(1):217–45.

30. Hurrell E, Kucerova E, Loughlin M, et al. Neonatal enteral feeding tubes as loci for colonisation by members of the Enterobacteriaceae. BMC Infect Dis 2009;9:146.
31. Mehall JR, Kite CA, Saltzman DA, et al. Prospective study of the incidence and complications of bacterial contamination of enteral feeding in neonates. J Pediatr Surg 2002;37:1177–82.
32. Christensen RD, Gordon PV, Besner GE. Can we cut the incidence of necrotizing enterocolitis in half–today? Fetal Pediatr Pathol 2010;29:185–98.
33. Patole SK, de Klerk N. Impact of standardised feeding regimens on incidence of neonatal necrotising enterocolitis: a systematic review and meta-analysis of observational studies. Arch Dis Child Fetal Neonatal Ed 2005;90:F147–51.
34. Lucas A, Cole TJ. Breast milk and necrotizing enterocolitis. Lancet 1990;336: 1519–23.
35. Gephart SM, Effken JA, McGrath JM, et al. Expert consensus building using e-Delphi for necrotizing enterocolitis risk assessment. J Obstet Gynecol Neonatal Nurs 2013;42:332–47.
36. Seigel JK, Tanaka DT, Goldberg RN, et al. Economic impact of human milk on medical charges of extremely low birth weight infants. Breastfeed Med 2014;9: 233–4.
37. Johnson TJ, Patel AL, Bigger HR, et al. Cost savings of human milk as a strategy to reduce the incidence of necrotizing enterocolitis in very low birth weight infants. Neonatology 2015;107:271–6.
38. Colaizy TT, Bartick MC, Jegier BJ, et al. Impact of optimized breastfeeding on the costs of necrotizing enterocolitis in extremely low birthweight infants. J Pediatr 2016;175:100–5.
39. Gephart SM, Hanson C, Wetzel CM, et al. NEC-zero recommendations from scoping review of evidence to prevent and foster timely recognition of necrotizing enterocolitis. Matern Health Neonatol Perinatol 2017;3:23.
40. Parker MG, Patel AL. Using quality improvement to increase human milk use for preterm infants. Semin Perinatol 2017;41:175–86.
41. Quigley M, Embleton ND, McGuire W. Formula versus donor breast milk for feeding preterm or low birth weight infants. Cochrane Database Syst Rev 2018;(6):CD002971.
42. Henderson G, Craig S, Brocklehurst P, et al. Enteral feeding regimens and necrotising enterocolitis in preterm infants: a multicentre case-control study. Arch Dis Child Fetal Neonatal Ed 2009;94(2):F120–3.
43. Jasani B, Patole S. Standardized feeding regimen for reducing necrotizing enterocolitis in preterm infants: an updated systematic review. J Perinatol 2017; 37:827–33.
44. Berseth CL. Neonatal small intestinal motility: motor responses to feeding in term and preterm infants. J Pediatr 1990;117:777–82.
45. Stoll B, Chang X, Fan MZ, et al. Enteral nutrient intake determines the rate of intestinal protein synthesis and accretion in neonatal pigs. Am J Physiol 2000;279: G288–94.
46. Burrin DG, Stoll B. Key nutrients and growth factors for the neonatal gastrointestinal tract. Clin Perinatol 2002;29:65–96.
47. Morgan J, Young L, McGuire W. Delayed introduction of progressive enteral feeds to prevent necrotising enterocolitis in very low birth weight infants. Cochrane Database Syst Rev 2014;(12):CD001970.
48. Hsieh EM, Hornik CP, Clark RH, et al. Medication use in the neonatal intensive care unit. Am J Perinatol 2014;31:811–21.

49. Esaiassen E, Fjalstad JW, Juvet LK, et al. Antibiotic exposure in neonates and early adverse outcomes: a systematic review and metaanalysis. J Antimicrob Chemother 2017;72:1858–70.

50. Fjalstad JW, Esaiassen E, Juvet LK, et al. Antibiotic therapy in neonates and impact on gut microbiota and antibiotic resistance development: a systematic review. J Antimicrob Chemother 2018;73:569–80.

51. Cotten CM, Taylor S, Stoll B, et al. Prolonged duration of initial empirical antibiotic treatment is associated with increased rates of necrotizing enterocolitis and death for extremely low birth weight infants. Pediatrics 2009;123:58–66.

52. Kuppala VS, Meinzen-Derr J, Morrow AL, et al. Prolonged initial empirical antibiotic treatment is associated with adverse outcomes in premature infants. J Pediatr 2011;159:720–5.

53. Alexander VN, Northrup V, Bizzarro MJ. Antibiotic exposure in the newborn intensive care unit and the risk of necrotizing enterocolitis. J Pediatr 2011;159:392–7.

54. Makri V, Davies G, Cannell S, et al. Managing antibiotics wisely: a quality improvement programme in a tertiary neonatal unit in the UK. BMJ Open Qual 2018;7:e000285.

55. Puopolo KM, Mukhopadhyay S, Hansen NI, et al. Identification of extremely premature infants at low risk for early-onset sepsis. Pediatrics 2017;140 [pii: e20170925].

56. Guillet R, Stoll BJ, Cotten CM, et al. Association of H2-blocker therapy and higher incidence of necrotizing enterocolitis in very low birth weight infants. Pediatrics 2006;117:e137–42.

57. Terrin G, Passariello A, De Curtis M, et al. Ranitidine is associated with infections, necrotizing enterocolitis, and fatal outcome in newborns. Pediatrics 2012;129: e40–5. Available at: www.pediatrics.org/cgi/content/full/129/1/e40pmid: 22157140.

58. Wheatley E, Kennedy KA. Cross-over trial of treatment for bradycardia attributed to gastroesophageal reflux in preterm infants. J Pediatr 2009;155:516–21.

59. Mohamed A, Shah PS. Transfusion associated necrotizing enterocolitis: a meta-analysis of observational data. Pediatrics 2012;129:529–40.

60. Hay S, Zupancic JA, Flannery DD, et al. Should we believe in transfusion-associated enterocolitis? Applying a GRADE to the literature. Semin Perinatol 2017;41:80–91.

61. Kirpalani H, Zupancic JA. Do transfusions cause necrotizing enterocolitis? Semin Perinatol 2012;36:269–76.

62. Maheshwari A, Patel RM, Christensen RD. Anemia, red blood cell transfusions, and necrotizing enterocolitis. Semin Pediatr Surg 2018;27:47–51.

63. Patel RM, Knezevic A, Shenvi N, et al. Association of red blood cell transfusion, anemia, and necrotizing enterocolitis in very low-birth-weight infants. JAMA 2016; 315:889–97.

64. Singh R, Visintainer ID, Frantz ID III, et al. Association of necrotizing enterocolitis with anemia and packed red blood cell transfusions in preterm infants. J Perinatol 2011;31:176–82.

65. Derienzo C, Smith PB, Tanaka D, et al. Feeding practices and other risk factors for developing transfusion-associated necrotizing enterocolitis. Early Hum Dev 2014;90:237–40.

66. Christensen RD, Lambert DK, Henry E, et al. Is "transfusion-associated necrotizing enterocolitis" an authentic pathogenic entity? Transfusion 2009;50: 1106–12.

67. Sharma R, Kraemer DF, Torrazza RM, et al. Packed red blood cell transfusion is not associated with increased risk of necrotizing enterocolitis in premature infants. J Perinatol 2014;34:858–62.

68. Le VT, Klebanoff MA, Talavera MM, et al. Transient effects of transfusion and feeding advances (volumetric and caloric) on necrotizing enterocolitis development: a case-crossover study. PLoS One 2017;12:e0179724.

69. El-Dib M, Narang S, Lee E, et al. Red blood cell transfusion, feeding and necrotizing enterocolitis in preterm infants. J Perinatol 2011;31:183–7.

70. Jasani B, Rao S, Patole S. Withholding feeds and transfusion-associated necrotizing enterocolitis in preterm infants: a systematic review. Adv Nutr 2017;8: 764–9.

Impact of Toll-Like Receptor 4 Signaling in Necrotizing Enterocolitis: The State of the Science

Belgacem Mihi, DVM, PhD[a], Misty Good, MD, MS[a,b],*

KEYWORDS

- Necrotizing enterocolitis • TLR4 • Inflammation • Epithelial cells

KEY POINTS

- Necrotizing enterocolitis (NEC) is a devastating gastrointestinal disease associated with microbial colonization of the immature intestine, which can result in an inappropriate immune response.
- The inflammatory response is partly due to the high expression of Toll-like receptor 4 (TLR4) in the intestine of premature infants.
- Exaggerated TLR4 signaling results in the impairment of the epithelial barrier.
- Inhibition of the TLR4-signaling pathway and its downstream targets can lead to reduced NEC severity and may translate into new drugs to treat and/or prevent NEC development.

INTRODUCTION

Since the emergence of early eukaryotic organisms, a plethora of sophisticated defense mechanisms has evolved to protect the host from invading pathogens and to ensure species survival.[1,2] A key feature of an optimal protective mechanism is the effective discrimination of harmful threats from innocuous and beneficial commensal entities.[3] Despite the high efficacy of the immune system in preventing deadly infections in adults, the morbidity inherent to infectious diseases is substantially higher in

Disclosure Statement: The authors have nothing to disclose and no conflicts of interest.
Funding Sources: M. Good is supported by grants K08DK101608 and R03DK111473 from the National Institutes of Health, March of Dimes Foundation Grant No. 5-FY17-79, and the Children's Discovery Institute of Washington University and St. Louis Children's Hospital.
a Division of Newborn Medicine, Department of Pediatrics, Washington University School of Medicine, 660 South Euclid Avenue, Campus Box 8208, St Louis, MO 63110, USA; b Department of Pathology and Immunology, Washington University School of Medicine, 660 South Euclid Avenue, Campus Box 8208, St Louis, MO 63110, USA
* Corresponding author. Division of Newborn Medicine, Department of Pediatrics, Washington University School of Medicine, St. Louis Children's Hospital, 660 South Euclid Avenue, Campus Box 8208, McDonnell Pediatric Research Building Office 4102, St Louis, MO 63110.
E-mail address: mistygood@wustl.edu

Clin Perinatol 46 (2019) 145–157
https://doi.org/10.1016/j.clp.2018.09.007
0095-5108/19/© 2018 Elsevier Inc. All rights reserved.

human neonates.[4,5] Furthermore, the prevalence of infections is significantly greater in preterm infants compared with term newborns.[6] Shortly after birth, the neonates experience a massive microbial colonization of their mucosal surfaces.[7] The early cross-talk between these microbial communities and the host is critical for the optimal development of host immunity.[8] This was evidenced by antibiotic treatment during infancy as well as the lack of microbial colonization in mice models leading to increased susceptibility to autoimmune and infectious diseases.[9–12] On the other hand, the bacterial colonization of the immature intestine of preterm infants is associated with the induction of a detrimental inflammatory response leading to the development of necrotizing enterocolitis (NEC).[13] NEC is a devastating gastrointestinal disease affecting up to 10% of premature infants with the highest incidence among those with a birth weight less than 1500 g and postmenstrual age of 32 weeks.[14–16] Although significant progress has been made in understanding of the molecular mechanisms behind the development of NEC, the optimal therapeutic strategies remain elusive.[17] Therefore, a better understanding of the developmental changes of the immune system during the neonatal period is required to implement new treatments to prevent the development of this devastating disease.

The immune surveillance of the host environment is carried out by pattern recognition receptors that play a central role in the first line of host defense. These receptors, which include Toll-like receptors (TLRs), retinoic acid–inducible gene-I–like receptors, nucleotide-binding oligomerization domain (NOD)-like receptors, and C-type lectin receptors, have the ability to recognize a wide range of intrinsic and extrinsic danger signals, namely pathogen-associated molecular patterns and danger-associated molecular patterns.[2] This article describes how the innate TLR response during early life correlates with the susceptibility of infants to inflammatory disorders, with a particular emphasis on the role of epithelial TLR4 in the initiation of the gastrointestinal disease NEC.

TOLL-LIKE RECEPTORS' FUNCTION IN THE HEMATOPOIETIC CELL COMPARTMENT DURING EARLY LIFE

TLRs are expressed by various types of hematopoietic and nonhematopoietic cells where they play a critical role in the induction of protective host immune responses as well as the development of detrimental inflammation.[2] In the hematopoietic cell compartment of neonates, TLRs and their downstream signaling molecules seem to be expressed at comparable levels to their adult counterparts.[18] Moreover, the peripheral blood monocytes can enhance the expression of TLRs in response to newborn sepsis, indicating that they are adequately expressed during infection.[19] Despite the normal expression levels of TLRs on newborn leukocytes, the cytokines produced on their activation differ drastically from those observed in adults. Intriguingly, TLR-mediated cytokine production is also distinct between preterm and term infants. TLR stimulation of preterm human blood leukocytes is characterized by high levels of interleukin (IL)-10, whereas IL-6 and IL-23 are the main landmarks of the term neonates' immune cells.[20–22] These patterns tend to change over the course of life toward tumor necrosis factor α and IL-1β production.[21] Furthermore, the poor TLR-mediated interferon response observed in the newborns evolves quickly during the first weeks of life to reach similar levels to those observed in adults.[21] The molecular basis of these differences is still not well understood. The weak interferon response during early life was attributed to the impaired nuclear translocation of interferon response factor 7.[23] Furthermore, newborn blood contains high amounts of adenosine compared with adult plasma.[24] Adenosine signals through adenosine receptors to generate cyclic adenosine monophosphate, which in turn can inhibit helper T-cell (T$_H$)1 differentiation while promoting IL-10, IL-6, and IL-23 production.[24–26] This pattern has a direct implication on vaccine responsiveness in neonates. In line with the anti-inflammatory cytokine production in preterm infants, several studies have highlighted the weak immune response induced by vaccines that were administered to preterm infants around birth whereas later vaccinations result in effective protection.[27,28] On the other hand, the exaggerated immune response after TLR stimulation in early life has been associated with a large panel of inflammatory disorders, including NEC, neonatal chronic lung disease, and periventricular white matter injury.[29,30] This seems to be in contradiction with the aforementioned regulatory cytokine profile in preterm immune cells, suggesting that the susceptibility of premature neonates to TLR-driven inflammation is at least partly initiated in the nonhematopoietic cell compartment.

EPITHELIAL TOLL-LIKE RECEPTOR 4 SIGNALING: A KEY FACTOR IN NECROTIZING ENTEROCOLITIS DEVELOPMENT

Over the past several years, considerable attention has been devoted to investigating the role of TLR4 signaling in the pathogenesis of NEC. This particular interest was motivated by early studies demonstrating that TLR2 and TLR4 are constitutively expressed by fetal enterocytes and that lipopolysaccharide (LPS) as well as IL-1B can modulate their expression.[31] Furthermore, TLR2, TLR4, and their related signaling molecules were shown to be highly expressed in fetal enterocytes compared with their mature adult counterparts. This differential expression was further evidenced in small intestinal cells during NEC, which are characterized by significantly higher expression of TLR4 than the healthy enterocytes.[32] Strikingly, it was shown that the cytosolic internalization of TLR4 is significantly higher in the mature intestinal cells suggesting that the excessive inflammatory response observed during NEC is at least partly due to the overexpression and the exaggerated activity of TLR4 in the preterm intestine.[32] These findings were further supported by the fact that LPS activation of TLR4 in intestinal cells is significantly higher in preterm mice compared with naturally delivered controls.[33] Importantly, the expression of TLR4 is substantially elevated during human NEC.[34] In an attempt to determine the molecular mechanism behind the high expression of TLR4 in preterm infants, a study performed by Soliman and colleagues[35] suggested that platelet-activating factor, initially incriminated in the development of NEC, is responsible for the overexpression of TLR4 in the premature intestine, thereby resulting in an exaggerated inflammation during NEC.[36] Other than the well-documented role of TLR4 in the activation of an inflammatory program in epithelial cells, it is also known to contribute to bacterial translocation across the mucosal barrier, which likely contributes to the development of the septic shock picture observed during NEC.[37] The functional evidence for the implication of TLR4 in the development of NEC came from the use of a murine model of the disease. Jilling and colleagues[38] as well as Hackam and colleagues[34,39] have shown that TLR4 is required for development of NEC through the impairment of the epithelial barrier integrity. Mechanistically, TLR4 can affect the homeostasis of the intestinal epithelium through different pathways. During intestinal injury, enterocyte migration throughout the crypt-villus axis can be affected by the activation of TLR4. This can be achieved by modulation of the cell-extracellular matrix interaction.[34,40] Unlike in the adult, TLR4 activation in the premature intestine is associated with the induction of an apoptotic program and the reduction of cell proliferation resulting in the impairment of epithelial cell regeneration[34,41,42] (**Fig. 1**). The stimulation of the TLR4 signaling cascade is associated with the induction of autophagy in epithelial cells, which has a negative impact on their migration during NEC.[43] Therefore, mice lacking the expression of the autophagy gene ATG7 were protected against NEC via the reduction of Ras homolog family member A (RhoA)-GTPase activation and subsequently, the enhancement of enterocyte migration. In line with these data, the expression levels of autophagy-related genes are relatively high in the premature intestine.[43] The role of TLR4-mediated inhibition of enterocyte migration was further evidenced in another study where the extracellular high-mobility group box 1 released during intestinal inflammation was found to enhance cell-matrix adhesiveness and to reduce enterocyte migration by the activating RhoA in a TLR4-dependent manner.[44] In parallel to the inhibition of cell migration, Sodhi and colleagues[42] showed that a TLR4-mediated reduction of epithelial cell proliferation is triggered by the activation of glycogen synthase kinase 3β and the reduction of β-catenin activity.[42] The coexpression of TLR4 and leucine-rich repeat-containing G-protein coupled receptor 5 (LGR5), an intestinal stem cell (ISC) marker, suggested that TLR4 regulation of the epithelial cell homeostasis could be driven by the activation of nuclear factor (NF)-κB in ISCs. Thus, TLR4 was found to promote the activation of p53 up-regulated modulator of apoptosis, which in turn prevents cell proliferation and initiates a cell death program.[41] A recent report has uncovered another mechanism by which TLR4 modulates ISC viability via the initiation of an endoplasmic reticulum (ER) stress during NEC.[45] The study revealed that TLR4 activation triggers ER stress in ISC by activating protein kinase-related PKR-like ER kinase (PERK) and C/EBP homologous protein (CHOP).[45] Moreover, genetic perturbation of PERK and CHOP conferred a significant protection against experimental murine

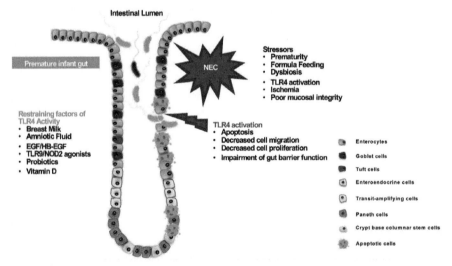

Fig. 1. Inhibition of TLR4 signaling as a potential strategy to cure/prevent the development of NEC. During the first days of life, several factors, such as formula feeding, high expression of TLR4, microbial colonization, and hypoxic stress, can trigger an inflammatory process leading to the development of NEC. Exaggerated TLR4 activity in the premature intestine plays a critical role in the pathogenesis of NEC by inducing epithelial cell apoptosis as well as reducing cell proliferation and cell migration throughout the crypt villi-axis. Altogether, these events lead to the impairment of the epithelial barrier integrity and the translocation of the luminal microorganisms which in turn initiate an exaggerated intestinal inflammatory response. Factors found in the breast milk and/or in amniotic fluid, including EGF/HB-EGF and vitamin D, have the ability to counteract the TLR4-mediated inflammation. In addition, probiotics can prevent the development of NEC by activating TLR9 and NOD2, dampening TLR4 signaling.

NEC.[45] Apart from the role of TLR4 in the modulation of the epithelial barrier integrity, it was shown to influence the differentiation of epithelial cells because mice deficient in TLR4 specifically in their intestinal epithelium are characterized by a marked increase in goblet cell number and mucin 2 expression.[46] The effect of decreased goblet cell number on NEC development in premature infants was evidenced by Sodhi and colleagues who demonstrated that the inhibition of γ-secretase and Notch signaling enhance goblet cell development, leading to a significant decrease in NEC susceptibility. In light of these findings, it is tempting to speculate that the increased differentiation of goblet cells on the ablation of the TLR4 gene and the resulting enhancement of antimicrobial peptide protection might explain the attenuated disease severity in these mice compared with their wild-type littermates.

Besides the critical role of TLR4 in the impairment of the epithelial integrity, a recent report has highlighted the role of TLR4 in the modulation of the CD4 T-cell response during NEC.[39] Similarly to inflammatory bowel disease in adults, NEC is associated with an intestinal T_H17/regulatory T-cell (Treg) imbalance.[39,47,48] In accordance with this observation, RAG knockout mice, which lack B-cell and T-cell repertoires, are protected from NEC.[39,49] Furthermore, Colliou and colleagues[50] have identified a commensal *Propionibacterium* strain named UF1 that has the ability to dampen the intestinal inflammation during NEC via the reduction of T_H17 cell expansion in the gut. Egan and colleagues[39] demonstrated that TLR4 activation in intestinal epithelial cells was responsible for the Treg/T_H7 imbalance through the up-regulation of CCR9/CCL25. Moreover, the TLR4-mediated T_H17 polarization during NEC was associated with the disruption of the epithelial barrier. Hence, the neutralization of IL-17 resulted in reduced NEC severity.[39]

As discussed previously, TLRs are expressed by different nonhematopoietic cells, including endothelial cells where they modulate their function on pathogen invasion and tissue damage.[51] It has long been believed that the impairment of the intestinal blood perfusion is a prerequisite for the development of intestinal injury and NEC in preterm infants.[52] Therefore, it was hypothesized that TLR4 activation specifically on the endothelial cell compartment is an important event preceding NEC development. This hypothesis was tested by Yazji and colleagues,[53] who investigated the impact of a specific deletion of the TLR4 locus in endothelial cells in a mouse model of NEC. They found that the absence of TLR4 expression in murine endothelial cells is associated with a significant reduction of NEC severity compared with endothelial TLR4 sufficient animals.[53] In addition, they showed that the stimulation of TLR4 in the endothelium is accompanied by reduced perfusion of the intestinal microvasculature. This impairment of the microvasculature perfusion was due to MyD-88–dependent reduction of endothelial nitric oxide synthase production.[53] These data further suggest that the absence of nitrate in infant formula might be the cause of impaired intestinal perfusion during NEC. As such, supplementation of infant formula with nitrate restored the intestinal perfusion and lead to a reduced disease severity in a neonatal mouse model of NEC.[53]

RESTRAINING FACTORS OF TOLL-LIKE RECEPTOR 4 ACTIVITY IN THE PREMATURE INTESTINE

Despite the experimental evidence attesting the central role of TLR4 in the development of NEC, only a fraction of premature infants are affected by NEC. This suggests the existence of physiologic processes that can counteract the deleterious effects of the high TLR4-mediated activity in the intestine of premature neonates. Several studies have shed light on different molecular mechanisms allowing the premature intestine to prevent the initiation of a harmful TLR4-mediated inflammation in the setting of NEC and are discussed in further detail.

TOLL-LIKE RECEPTOR 9 AND NUCLEOTIDE-BINDING OLIGOMERIZATION DOMAIN-CONTAINING PROTEIN 2

By extending the investigation to the other pattern recognition receptors, TLR9 and NOD2 were identified as potent inhibitors of TLR4 signaling, thus preventing the development of NEC. Unlike TLR4, which recognizes bacterial LPS, TLR9 has the ability to recognize and to interact with microbial unmethylated CpG DNA motifs.[54] The apical TLR9 activation prevents the subsequent TLR4-induced inflammation by inhibiting NF-κB signaling.[55] Furthermore, TLR9 deficient mice are more susceptible to colonic inflammation than their wild littermates.[55] A time course study revealed that the high TLR4 expression in embryonic murine intestine drastically decreases around delivery, whereas TLR9 expression follows an opposite pattern, suggesting that the intestinal TLR4/TLR9 balance might determine the susceptibility of the premature intestine to NEC.[56] In agreement with these findings and by contrast to TLR4, TLR9 expression in the intestines of human infants with NEC is significantly lower in comparison with controls.[56,57] Moreover, the reduced incidence of NEC on TLR9 stimulation was attributed to the inhibition of TLR4 activity through the localization of IL-1 receptor-associated kinase-M (IRAK-M) in the Golgi apparatus.[56] In a recent report, Good et al. demonstrated that the protection conferred by *Lactobacillus rhamnosus* HN001 and its microbial DNA against NEC is achieved by the inhibition of TLR4 in a TLR9-dependent manner.[58]

In addition to TLR9, it seemed intuitive to explore the implication of NOD-containing protein 2 (NOD2) in the pathogenesis of NEC given its established role in adult inflammatory bowel disease.[59] Thus, the genetic analysis performed in a population of infants with a very low birth weight revealed that the accumulation of 2 or more genetic variants in NOD2 alleles was associated with a high risk of NEC development requiring surgical intervention.[60] Similarly, Richardson and colleagues[61] have shown that NOD2 reduces the susceptibility to NEC in mice through the inhibition of TLR4 signaling in enterocytes. The authors found that the activation of NOD2 resulted in the repression of second mitochondria-derived activator of caspases (SMAC), which in turn leads to reduced enterocyte apoptosis and the enhancement of the mucosal barrier integrity.[61] Strikingly, it was recently shown that NOD2 could sense the intensity of TLR4 activity in macrophages and can modulate the resulting IL-12 expression.[62] Under intense TLR4 signaling, NOD2 can repress IL-12 expression whereas poor TLR4 signaling can switch NOD2 activity toward a synergic stimulation of IL-12 production.[62] The balance of NOD2 activity in macrophages is regulated by receptor-interacting serine/threonine kinase 2 and the transcriptional regulator CCAAT/enhancer-binding protein α.[62] The existence of such regulatory mechanisms in epithelial cells remains, however, unknown.

HEAT SHOCK PROTEIN 70

During heat stress, cells can respond to the deleterious aggregation of unfolded proteins by enhancing the expression of a large panel of protective factors referred to as heat shock proteins (HSPs).[63] HSP70, a member of the heat stress protein family, displays a cytoprotective role in intestinal epithelial cells.[64–66] HSP70 expression in epithelial cells can be triggered by several factors including intestinal microbiota and cytokines. Moreover, HSP70 is induced by breast milk to promote the maintenance of the epithelial barrier in rat immature intestine.[67] Accordingly, the low expression of HSP70 was associated with the development of NEC.[68] From the molecular perspective, TLR4 signaling is restrained by HSP70 via a co-chaperone E3 Ub ligase carboxyl terminus of the Hsc70-interacting protein (CHIP)-mediated ubiquitination and degradation of TLR4 that required a functional EEVD-binding domain in the C-terminus of HSP70.[68] Hence, HSP70 deficiency leads to enhanced disease severity in a murine NEC model, whereas the overexpression or the chemical induction of HSP70 protect against NEC.[68]

BREAST MILK AND AMNIOTIC FLUID

It is widely accepted that breastfeeding is critical in shaping the newborn immune system and providing protection against infections and inflammatory disorders later in life.[69] In the context of NEC, breast milk administration is associated with a lower incidence of the disease suggesting the existence of protective components of breast milk that can potentially be used in new therapeutic approaches.[70,71] In the same manner, the authors' work revealed that breast milk protects against the development of NEC in murine pups.[72] This protection was abolished by removing epidermal growth factor (EGF) from the breast milk, indicating that this growth factor is necessary to protect the intestine of premature infant against NEC. Similarly, heparin-binding EGF-like growth factor (HB-EGF) was shown to prevent the development of NEC in neonatal rats.[73,74] These data were further supported as mice lacking the expression of EGF receptor (EGFR) in their intestinal epithelium were not protected against NEC with breast milk.[72] Therefore, genetic polymorphism analysis of the EGFR locus in infants with NEC is of great interest. Additional studies revealed that the EGF contained in breast milk prevents NEC development likely via the inhibition of TLR4-induced epithelial cell death and by promoting the regeneration of the mucosal barrier by stimulating enterocyte proliferation.[72] Moreover, they showed that the inhibition of TLR4 activation by breast milk is achieved by the suppression of Glycogen synthase kinase 3β (GSK3β) activity in enterocytes.[72]

Similarly to breast milk, amniotic fluid contains several immunomodulatory and antimicrobial factors, which can improve the mucosal barrier integrity in the setting of intestinal inflammation.[75] To explore the effect of amniotic fluid on gut inflammation, newborn rats were injected with amniotic fluid stem cells and subjected to experimental NEC.[76] The animals, which received amniotic fluid stem cells, displayed reduced NEC incidence and enhanced epithelial cell regeneration. The beneficial effect of amniotic fluid was ascribed to an augmented expression of cyclooxygenase 2 in stromal cells.[76] It was also suggested that the protective function of cyclooxygenase-2 might be due to an indirect activation of EGFR.[76] In another study, the authors have shown that the reduction of epithelial EGFR expression was associated increased susceptibility to NEC in mice and humans.[77] Similarly to breast milk, the authors found that amniotic fluid dampens TLR4-mediated inflammation through the activation of EGFR signaling in neonatal intestine.[77] This was consistent with the absence of amniotic fluid protection in the mice lacking the expression of EGFR in intestinal epithelial cells.[77] It is worth mentioning that breast milk of mothers giving birth to extremely premature infants is significantly enriched in EGF, suggesting that at least some of the premature infants have defective EGFR signaling.[78]

VITAMIN D

Vitamin D is a fat-soluble vitamin with a large spectrum of biological activities.[79] In the liver, vitamin D is transformed into 1,25-dihydroxyvitamin D, an active metabolite that signals through vitamin D receptor.[79] Vitamin D plays an important role in regulating both innate and adaptive immune responses.[80] For example, it was shown that vitamin D deficiency was positively correlated with the severity of human as well as murine inflammatory bowel disease.[81–83] Consistently, in vivo and in vitro data demonstrated that vitamin D promotes epithelial cell migration and the enhancement of tight junctions.[83] In addition, vitamin D vitiates NF-κB signaling, resulting in reduced epithelial cell death.[82] Similarly, a low level of maternal/neonatal 1,25-dihydroxyvitamin D was shown to be a risk for NEC development.[84,85] In accordance with the protective role of vitamin D in the context of adult inflammatory bowel disease, Shi and colleagues[85] have found that vitamin D treatment significantly attenuates NEC severity in a rat model. They also and found that vitamin D significantly repressed TLR4 expression, while promoting the expression of tight junction proteins and dampening epithelial cell apoptosis.

SUMMARY

Despite the recent advances in understanding of the pathophysiology of NEC, the translation into an effective therapy has yet to occur, and the mortality caused by this disease in the premature infants remains high. As discussed previously, TLR4 signaling plays a central role in the induction of NEC through the modulation of the epithelial cell barrier and the regulation of the innate and adaptive immune responses. Therefore, TLR4 inhibition seems to be a promising target for new drug development and it is the authors' hope that one day this devastating consequence of prematurity can be prevented.

Best practices

What is the current practice?

- NEC is a common gastrointestinal disease with a high mortality rate that affects premature infants.
- Risk factors for NEC include prematurity, microbial colonization, and lack of breast milk feedings.
- NEC involves an exaggerated immune response in the setting of elevated expression of TLR4, leading to necrosis of the epithelial barrier.
- Currently, there is no effective treatment or optimal therapeutic strategy to prevent NEC.

What changes in current practice are likely to improve outcomes?

- Prioritizing human milk feedings can decrease the risk of NEC in premature infants.
- Several potential TLR4 signaling-related molecules have been identified as potential targets to identify infants at the highest risk for NEC and to develop novel therapeutics.

Summary statement

- NEC is a devastating consequence of prematurity and microbial imbalance in the intestine. The use of preclinical animal models has identified potential new therapeutic strategies that could be translated into clinical trials in the near future.

REFERENCES

1. Zhang Q, Zmasek CM, Godzik A. Domain architecture evolution of pattern-recognition receptors. Immunogenetics 2010;62(5):263–72.
2. Takeuchi O, Akira S. Pattern recognition receptors and inflammation. Cell 2010; 140(6):805–20.

3. Chu H, Mazmanian SK. Innate immune recognition of the microbiota promotes host-microbial symbiosis. Nat Immunol 2013;14(7):668–75.

4. Torow N, Marsland BJ, Hornef MW, et al. Neonatal mucosal immunology. Mucosal Immunol 2017;10(1):5–17.

5. Kollmann TR, Kampmann B, Mazmanian SK, et al. Protecting the newborn and young infant from infectious diseases: lessons from immune ontogeny. Immunity 2017;46(3):350–63.

6. Jiang Z, Ye GY. 1:4 matched case-control study on influential factor of early onset neonatal sepsis. Eur Rev Med Pharmacol Sci 2013;17(18):2460–6.

7. Gritz EC, Bhandari V. The human neonatal gut microbiome: a brief review. Front Pediatr 2015;3:17.

8. Tanaka M, Nakayama J. Development of the gut microbiota in infancy and its impact on health in later life. Allergol Int 2017;66(4):515–22.

9. Miyoshi J, Bobe AM, Miyoshi S, et al. Peripartum antibiotics promote gut dysbiosis, loss of immune tolerance, and inflammatory bowel disease in genetically prone offspring. Cell Rep 2017;20(2):491–504.

10. Bouskra D, Brezillon C, Berard M, et al. Lymphoid tissue genesis induced by commensals through NOD1 regulates intestinal homeostasis. Nature 2008; 456(7221):507–10.

11. Hall JA, Bouladoux N, Sun CM, et al. Commensal DNA limits regulatory T cell conversion and is a natural adjuvant of intestinal immune responses. Immunity 2008; 29(4):637–49.

12. Kronman MP, Zaoutis TE, Haynes K, et al. Antibiotic exposure and IBD development among children: a population-based cohort study. Pediatrics 2012;130(4): e794–803.

13. La Rosa PS, Warner BB, Zhou Y, et al. Patterned progression of bacterial populations in the premature infant gut. Proc Natl Acad Sci U S A 2014;111(34): 12522–7.

14. Yee WH, Soraisham AS, Shah VS, et al. Incidence and timing of presentation of necrotizing enterocolitis in preterm infants. Pediatrics 2012;129(2):e298–304.

15. Stoll BJ, Hansen NI, Bell EF, et al. Trends in care practices, morbidity, and mortality of extremely preterm neonates, 1993-2012. JAMA 2015;314(10):1039–51.

16. Sharma R, Hudak ML. A clinical perspective of necrotizing enterocolitis: past, present, and future. Clin Perinatol 2013;40(1):27–51.

17. Neu J, Walker WA. Necrotizing enterocolitis. N Engl J Med 2011;364(3):255–64.

18. Dasari P, Zola H, Nicholson IC. Expression of Toll-like receptors by neonatal leukocytes. Pediatr Allergy Immunol 2011;22(2):221–8.

19. Zhang JP, Yang Y, Levy O, et al. Human neonatal peripheral blood leukocytes demonstrate pathogen-specific coordinate expression of TLR2, TLR4/MD2, and MyD88 during bacterial infection in vivo. Pediatr Res 2010;68(6):479–83.

20. Lavoie PM, Huang Q, Jolette E, et al. Profound lack of interleukin (IL)-12/IL-23p40 in neonates born early in gestation is associated with an increased risk of sepsis. J Infect Dis 2010;202(11):1754–63.

21. Corbett NP, Blimkie D, Ho KC, et al. Ontogeny of Toll-like receptor mediated cytokine responses of human blood mononuclear cells. PLoS One 2010;5(11): e15041.

22. Kollmann TR, Crabtree J, Rein-Weston A, et al. Neonatal innate TLR-mediated responses are distinct from those of adults. J Immunol 2009;183(11):7150–60.

23. Danis B, George TC, Goriely S, et al. Interferon regulatory factor 7-mediated responses are defective in cord blood plasmacytoid dendritic cells. Eur J Immunol 2008;38(2):507–17.

24. Levy O, Coughlin M, Cronstein BN, et al. The adenosine system selectively inhibits TLR-mediated TNF-alpha production in the human newborn. J Immunol 2006;177(3):1956–66.

25. Drygiannakis I, Ernst PB, Lowe D, et al. Immunological alterations mediated by adenosine during host-microbial interactions. Immunol Res 2011;50(1):69–77.

26. Power Coombs MR, Belderbos ME, Gallington LC, et al. Adenosine modulates Toll-like receptor function: basic mechanisms and translational opportunities. Expert Rev Anti Infect Ther 2011;9(2):261–9.

27. Esposito S, Serra D, Gualtieri L, et al. Vaccines and preterm neonates: why, when, and with what. Early Hum Dev 2009;85(10 Suppl):S43–5.

28. Baxter D. Impaired functioning of immune defenses to infection in premature and term infants and their implications for vaccination. Hum Vaccin 2010;6(6): 494–505.

29. Volpe JJ. Postnatal sepsis, necrotizing entercolitis, and the critical role of systemic inflammation in white matter injury in premature infants. J Pediatr 2008; 153(2):160–3.

30. Pryhuber GS. Postnatal infections and immunology affecting chronic lung disease of prematurity. Clin Perinatol 2015;42(4):697–718.

31. Fusunyan RD, Nanthakumar NN, Baldeon ME, et al. Evidence for an innate immune response in the immature human intestine: toll-like receptors on fetal enterocytes. Pediatr Res 2001;49(4):589–93.

32. Nanthakumar N, Meng D, Goldstein AM, et al. The mechanism of excessive intestinal inflammation in necrotizing enterocolitis: an immature innate immune response. PLoS One 2011;6(3):e17776.

33. Lotz M, Gutle D, Walther S, et al. Postnatal acquisition of endotoxin tolerance in intestinal epithelial cells. J Exp Med 2006;203(4):973–84.

34. Leaphart CL, Cavallo J, Gribar SC, et al. A critical role for TLR4 in the pathogenesis of necrotizing enterocolitis by modulating intestinal injury and repair. J Immunol 2007;179(7):4808–20.

35. Soliman A, Michelsen KS, Karahashi H, et al. Platelet-activating factor induces TLR4 expression in intestinal epithelial cells: implication for the pathogenesis of necrotizing enterocolitis. PLoS One 2010;5(10):e15044.

36. Caplan MS, Sun XM, Hsueh W. Hypoxia causes ischemic bowel necrosis in rats: the role of platelet-activating factor (PAF-acether). Gastroenterology 1990;99(4): 979–86.

37. Neal MD, Leaphart C, Levy R, et al. Enterocyte TLR4 mediates phagocytosis and translocation of bacteria across the intestinal barrier. J Immunol 2006;176(5): 3070–9.

38. Jilling T, Simon D, Lu J, et al. The roles of bacteria and TLR4 in rat and murine models of necrotizing enterocolitis. J Immunol 2006;177(5):3273–82.

39. Egan CE, Sodhi CP, Good M, et al. Toll-like receptor 4-mediated lymphocyte influx induces neonatal necrotizing enterocolitis. J Clin Invest 2016;126(2):495–508.

40. Qureshi FG, Leaphart C, Cetin S, et al. Increased expression and function of integrins in enterocytes by endotoxin impairs epithelial restitution. Gastroenterology 2005;128(4):1012–22.

41. Neal MD, Sodhi CP, Jia H, et al. Toll-like receptor 4 is expressed on intestinal stem cells and regulates their proliferation and apoptosis via the p53 up-regulated modulator of apoptosis. J Biol Chem 2012;287(44):37296–308.

42. Sodhi CP, Shi XH, Richardson WM, et al. Toll-like receptor-4 inhibits enterocyte proliferation via impaired beta-catenin signaling in necrotizing enterocolitis. Gastroenterology 2010;138(1):185–96.

43. Neal MD, Sodhi CP, Dyer M, et al. A critical role for TLR4 induction of autophagy in the regulation of enterocyte migration and the pathogenesis of necrotizing enterocolitis. J Immunol 2013;190(7):3541–51.

44. Dai S, Sodhi C, Cetin S, et al. Extracellular high mobility group box-1 (HMGB1) inhibits enterocyte migration via activation of Toll-like receptor-4 and increased cell-matrix adhesiveness. J Biol Chem 2010;285(7):4995–5002.

45. Afrazi A, Branca MF, Sodhi CP, et al. Toll-like receptor 4-mediated endoplasmic reticulum stress in intestinal crypts induces necrotizing enterocolitis. J Biol Chem 2014;289(14):9584–99.

46. Sodhi CP, Neal MD, Siggers R, et al. Intestinal epithelial Toll-like receptor 4 regulates goblet cell development and is required for necrotizing enterocolitis in mice. Gastroenterology 2012;143(3):708–18.e5.

47. Weitkamp JH, Koyama T, Rock MT, et al. Necrotising enterocolitis is characterised by disrupted immune regulation and diminished mucosal regulatory (FOXP3)/effector (CD4, CD8) T cell ratios. Gut 2013;62(1):73–82.

48. Pang Y, Du X, Xu X, et al. Monocyte activation and inflammation can exacerbate Treg/Th17 imbalance in infants with neonatal necrotizing enterocolitis. Int Immunopharmacol 2018;59:354–60.

49. He YM, Li X, Perego M, et al. Transitory presence of myeloid-derived suppressor cells in neonates is critical for control of inflammation. Nat Med 2018;24(2):224–31.

50. Colliou N, Ge Y, Sahay B, et al. Commensal Propionibacterium strain UF1 mitigates intestinal inflammation via Th17 cell regulation. J Clin Invest 2017;127(11):3970–86.

51. Salvador B, Arranz A, Francisco S, et al. Modulation of endothelial function by Toll like receptors. Pharmacol Res 2016;108:46–56.

52. Watkins DJ, Besner GE. The role of the intestinal microcirculation in necrotizing enterocolitis. Semin Pediatr Surg 2013;22(2):83–7.

53. Yazji I, Sodhi CP, Lee EK, et al. Endothelial TLR4 activation impairs intestinal microcirculatory perfusion in necrotizing enterocolitis via eNOS-NO-nitrite signaling. Proc Natl Acad Sci U S A 2013;110(23):9451–6.

54. Hemmi H, Takeuchi O, Kawai T, et al. A Toll-like receptor recognizes bacterial DNA. Nature 2000;408(6813):740–5.

55. Lee J, Mo JH, Katakura K, et al. Maintenance of colonic homeostasis by distinctive apical TLR9 signalling in intestinal epithelial cells. Nat Cell Biol 2006;8(12):1327–36.

56. Gribar SC, Sodhi CP, Richardson WM, et al. Reciprocal expression and signaling of TLR4 and TLR9 in the pathogenesis and treatment of necrotizing enterocolitis. J Immunol 2009;182(1):636–46.

57. Yin Y, Liu F, Li Y, et al. mRNA expression of TLR4, TLR9 and NF-kappaB in a neonatal murine model of necrotizing enterocolitis. Mol Med Rep 2016;14(3):1953–6.

58. Good M, Sodhi CP, Ozolek JA, et al. Lactobacillus rhamnosus HN001 decreases the severity of necrotizing enterocolitis in neonatal mice and preterm piglets: evidence in mice for a role of TLR9. Am J Physiol Gastrointest Liver Physiol 2014;306(11):G1021–32.

59. Eckmann L, Karin M. NOD2 and Crohn's disease: loss or gain of function? Immunity 2005;22(6):661–7.

60. Hartel C, Hartz A, Pagel J, et al. NOD2 loss-of-function mutations and risks of necrotizing enterocolitis or focal intestinal perforation in very low-birth-weight infants. Inflamm Bowel Dis 2016;22(2):249–56.

61. Richardson WM, Sodhi CP, Russo A, et al. Nucleotide-binding oligomerization domain-2 inhibits toll-like receptor-4 signaling in the intestinal epithelium. Gastroenterology 2010;139(3):904–17, 917 e1-6.
62. Kim H, Zhao Q, Zheng H, et al. A novel crosstalk between TLR4- and NOD2-mediated signaling in the regulation of intestinal inflammation. Sci Rep 2015;5: 12018.
63. Richter K, Haslbeck M, Buchner J. The heat shock response: life on the verge of death. Mol Cell 2010;40(2):253–66.
64. Hu S, Zhu X, Triggs JR, et al. Inflammation-induced, 3'UTR-dependent translational inhibition of Hsp70 mRNA impairs intestinal homeostasis. Am J Physiol Gastrointest Liver Physiol 2009;296(5):G1003–11.
65. Musch MW, Sugi K, Straus D, et al. Heat-shock protein 72 protects against oxidant-induced injury of barrier function of human colonic epithelial Caco2/bbe cells. Gastroenterology 1999;117(1):115–22.
66. Kojima K, Musch MW, Ren H, et al. Enteric flora and lymphocyte-derived cytokines determine expression of heat shock proteins in mouse colonic epithelial cells. Gastroenterology 2003;124(5):1395–407.
67. Liedel JL, Guo Y, Yu Y, et al. Mother's milk-induced Hsp70 expression preserves intestinal epithelial barrier function in an immature rat pup model. Pediatr Res 2011;69(5 Pt 1):395–400.
68. Afrazi A, Sodhi CP, Good M, et al. Intracellular heat shock protein-70 negatively regulates TLR4 signaling in the newborn intestinal epithelium. J Immunol 2012; 188(9):4543–57.
69. Newburg DS, Walker WA. Protection of the neonate by the innate immune system of developing gut and of human milk. Pediatr Res 2007;61(1):2–8.
70. Barlow B. Letter: necrotizing enterocolitis: protective factor in breast milk. N Engl J Med 1976;294(15):844–5.
71. Lucas A, Cole TJ. Breast milk and neonatal necrotising enterocolitis. Lancet 1990; 336(8730):1519–23.
72. Good M, Sodhi CP, Egan CE, et al. Breast milk protects against the development of necrotizing enterocolitis through inhibition of Toll-like receptor 4 in the intestinal epithelium via activation of the epidermal growth factor receptor. Mucosal Immunol 2015;8(5):1166–79.
73. Feng J, Besner GE. Heparin-binding epidermal growth factor-like growth factor promotes enterocyte migration and proliferation in neonatal rats with necrotizing enterocolitis. J Pediatr Surg 2007;42(1):214–20.
74. Yu X, Radulescu A, Zorko N, et al. Heparin-binding EGF-like growth factor increases intestinal microvascular blood flow in necrotizing enterocolitis. Gastroenterology 2009;137(1):221–30.
75. Dasgupta S, Jain SK. Protective effects of amniotic fluid in the setting of necrotizing enterocolitis. Pediatr Res 2017;82(4):584–95.
76. Zani A, Cananzi M, Fascetti-Leon F, et al. Amniotic fluid stem cells improve survival and enhance repair of damaged intestine in necrotising enterocolitis via a COX-2 dependent mechanism. Gut 2014;63(2):300–9.
77. Good M, Siggers RH, Sodhi CP, et al. Amniotic fluid inhibits Toll-like receptor 4 signaling in the fetal and neonatal intestinal epithelium. Proc Natl Acad Sci U S A 2012;109(28):11330–5.
78. Dvorak B, Fituch CC, Williams CS, et al. Increased epidermal growth factor levels in human milk of mothers with extremely premature infants. Pediatr Res 2003; 54(1):15–9.

79. Bouillon R, Carmeliet G, Verlinden L, et al. Vitamin D and human health: lessons from vitamin D receptor null mice. Endocr Rev 2008;29(6):726–76.

80. Sun J. Vitamin D and mucosal immune function. Curr Opin Gastroenterol 2010; 26(6):591–5.

81. Cantorna MT, Munsick C, Bemiss C, et al. 1,25-Dihydroxycholecalciferol prevents and ameliorates symptoms of experimental murine inflammatory bowel disease. J Nutr 2000;130(11):2648–52.

82. Liu W, Chen Y, Golan MA, et al. Intestinal epithelial vitamin D receptor signaling inhibits experimental colitis. J Clin Invest 2013;123(9):3983–96.

83. Kong J, Zhang Z, Musch MW, et al. Novel role of the vitamin D receptor in maintaining the integrity of the intestinal mucosal barrier. Am J Physiol Gastrointest Liver Physiol 2008;294(1):G208–16.

84. Cetinkaya M, Erener-Ercan T, Kalayci-Oral T, et al. Maternal/neonatal vitamin D deficiency: a new risk factor for necrotizing enterocolitis in preterm infants? J Perinatol 2017;37(6):673–8.

85. Shi Y, Liu T, Zhao X, et al. Vitamin D ameliorates neonatal necrotizing enterocolitis via suppressing TLR4 in a murine model. Pediatr Res 2018;83(5):1024–30.

Printed and bound by CPI Group (UK) Ltd, Croydon, CR0 4YY

03/10/2024

01040479-0014